CAN HOSPITALS SURVIVE?
The new competitive health care market

Jeff Charles Goldsmith

Can hospitals survive?

The new competitive
health care market

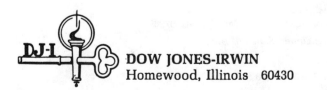

DOW JONES-IRWIN
Homewood, Illinois 60430

ISBN 0-87094-248-4
Library of Congress Catalog Card No. 81–67969

Printed in the United States of America

1 2 3 4 5 6 7 8 9 0 K 8 7 6 5 4 3 2 1

This book is dedicated to my sons, Jason and Trevor,
and to a healthy future for their children.

Foreword

This book is about the transition of the current organization of health services, from autonomous hospitals and physicians to corporate structures rivalling those in industry and business. The cottage industry of autonomous physicians in solo practice is developing into a complex network of referral relationships and, increasingly, group practices. The culmination of this evolution may be large scale prepaid group practices serving a known population.

Hospitals have likewise been enmeshed in the same web of developments as more capital and operating funds have been needed for modern operation. Physician-entrepreneurs created models of integrated hospital practice in the Mayo, Lahey, Ochsner and Cleveland clinics, which were organized around group practices of salaried physicians who billed on a fee-for-service basis. Later, well-known group practice prepayment plans, such as Kaiser Permanente, emerged in parts of the country. However, Blue Cross, Blue Shield, and private insurance companies helped to perpetuate the solo-practice, fee-for-service model. As the economy tightens, though, the government programs of Medicaid and Medicare as well as private insurers are looking for more structured service modes to help rationalize and contain the rising cost of personal health services.

The total health services enterprise in the United States gathers in more than $220 billion a year, around $1,000 for every person in the country. Many health services organizations now have individual cash flows in excess of $100 million annually. Health care is a large scale enterprise. Regulatory and planning agencies, as well as the third-party payers mentioned above, are trying to slow the pace of increase in expenditures by controlling supply and price, by deemphasizing institutional health services and directing more money to out-of-hospital services. No matter how remote, some form of universal national health insurance, whether through past models or some new form of competitive health care model, seems to hover in the background as a threat for increasing control by the third-party payer. Public demand for health care continues unabated. As sources of health funding tighten, this vast and seemingly inchoate enterprise called health services will require more skillful management.

This country has an entrepreneurial tradition which has spilled over from the private sector into health services. The professional and managerial corps in hospitals and related health agencies is both more numerous and better trained than in any country in the world. Still, are there enough managers with the entrepreneurial attitude and skills to continue to foster the dynamism in health services in this country as a countervailing force to increasing regulatory control by government? Will management settle for a fairly adequate but humdrum level of operation and innovation such as is occurring in other countries, or will it build on the American entrepreneurial tradition? Can management in health enterprises reach out both to serve and to sell what people want in response to their needs and financial resources? Can management move from a cottage industry mentality to an entrepreneurial mentality which will preserve the one on one relationship of physician to patient—the virtue of the cottage industry mode—within more complex structures? The awareness and influence of consumers is sure to increase. Can management tap their influence constructively?

This book by Dr. Jeff Goldsmith lays the groundwork for challenge to management in the health services in the future. The health services infrastructure is in place; good management can keep it moving forward. Let us hope that management will not be paralyzed by the many external forces which, at this point, seem intent only upon containing costs with whatever means possible with no clear idea of the consequences for the future condition of the health services, let alone peoples' health. This book is a beginning to comprehending the problem of managing in this difficult future and suggests directions for future strategies.

Odin W. Anderson
Professor of Sociology
Center for Health Administration Studies
University of Chicago

Preface

Even though it is early in the decade, it appears that competition will be a central concern of health professionals and policymakers during the 1980s. American society is rapidly nearing, or has already reached, the point where it is unwilling to commit the level of resources to health care that it has during the past 25 years. Health policy analysts have suggested that there are two paths toward a more sparing use of social resources for health care: increased regulation or increased competition. Past regulatory efforts seem to have failed to stem rising health care costs, and the political constituency for it is rapidly dwindling. Most commentators seem increasingly dubious about the ability of government to produce the economies needed.

The alternative path, increased competition, is a largely unknown quantity. Foremost among its advocates are articulate spokesmen for the health maintenance organization (HMO), such as Paul Ellwood, Jr. and Walter McClure of *Interstudy,* and the eminent social analyst, Alain Enthoven. These analysts have captured the imagination of influential members of Congress and the new administration in Washington. The competition they seek is between health *insurance* systems, including many possible variations upon the HMO, which seem to be able to make more efficient use of health services. Enthoven and his colleagues argue that competition between health care plans will help create a leaner health care system and reduce increases in health costs.

Thus most of the focus of the health policy debate over competition has been upon the insurance system, not on the physicians, hospitals, nursing homes, and other actors who deliver health care. How competition between health plans will affect the behavior of the delivery system itself is an issue which has yet to be aired in detail. The response of the managers and professionals to proposed procompetitive changes in the insurance system will determine the efficacy of competition as a mechanism for containing health care costs.

Those who have written about encouraging competition often begin by asserting how little competition there is in the health care system. While this may be true of conventional price competition in such heavily insured areas as inpatient hospital care, physicians and health care managers know that the health care market is already intensely competitive. It is naive to view competition as something that policymakers will inject into the health system; it is already a major feature of that system. Redirecting that competition to the nation's broader economic interests is the real task of the policymaker, a task which, given recent past history, is likely to be much more difficult and painful than anyone currently understands.

The underlying assumptions of competition advocates is that competing health care plans will begin to exert increasing market power in attempting to make efficient use of limited health care dollars. Health care financing will move away from cost and fee-for-service reimbursement and toward brokering of care for large and small groups of patients. To do this efficiently, plan managers will force tradeoffs among various modes of rendering care to minimize cost.

Exerting this purchasing power in the health care market will increasingly inject economic factors into the mediating role currently played by the patient's physician in deciding which procedures, and which facilities, to use to resolve the patient's medical problem. Health insurers will become more selective about the procedures and settings for which they are willing to reimburse, hedging upon the nearly absolute freedom of choice provided the physician by the current insurance system.

Rather than triggering reflexive opposition from the health care industry, proposals such as Enthoven's have received interested, even enthusiastic, receptions from industry leaders chafing under excessive government regulation, but also awakening to their increasing vulnerability in the competition for social resources. As a broad concept, competition resonates well with certain basic American values, such as free enterprise and entrepreneurship.

What is not fully appreciated by those who embrace competition is that it will mean a major restructuring of the health care industry and the demise of many existing institutions. Hundreds of hospitals will likely close their doors and as many as several thousand more may be acquired by large hospital management firms, as freestanding units become increasingly unable to compete effectively in price or quality of care. Physicians who have enjoyed unprecedented economic freedom face the prospect of declining incomes and an escalating threat to fee-for-service practice from prepaid health plans and integrated health care providers. Nursing homes will face an increasing array of noninstitutional health services for the elderly and chronically ill and a marked reduction in the rate of increase in social spending for institutional long-term care. Changing patterns of demand will pose a serious economic threat to many existing providers of health care, and force them to confront a changing world with new strategies for meeting peoples' health needs. There can be no true competition without economic risk. The society must be prepared to accommodate the failure of the inefficient or unresponsive health care providers.

The purpose of this book is to examine the competitive framework within which health care is provided in the United

States, with a view toward describing the transformation which increased economic competition is likely to work upon it. This book is not a policy analysis; many excellent works in this area already exist. Rather it is a strategic analysis of the impact of impending policy developments and a climate of increasing economic scarcity upon the structure and operations of the health care system.

For purposes of analysis and informed speculation, it will be assumed that through a series of incremental policy changes in both the public and private sectors there will be increased use of medical purchasing power. At the same time, given the nation's changing economic priorities, it is reasonable to assume that public outlays for health care will be systematically restrained over the next several years. Beyond the view that competition is, generically, a good thing, we will not advocate a particular approach to encouraging constructive economic competition in the health care industry. Rather it will be assumed that, whether through fiscal retrenchment by government, restructuring of health insurance plans, or both, economic pressures on all health care providers will increase. How these pressures will alter the incentives for physicians and health care managers is what this book intends to explore.

In order to do this, it is necessary to describe the principal features of the health care market today—its principal segments and the growth rates and factors associated with them. Since the hospital is the core institutional provider of health care, we will present a model of the health care market built around the demand for inpatient hospital services. This model will serve as a basis for exploring the economic trade-offs within the health care industry.

Having laid out the competitive framework in the health care system, the book will present some perspectives and strategies for surviving in the tightening health care market. It will explore the strategic response of corporations to tightening markets and relate these strategies and the structural changes they compel to health care institutions. Its analysis will stop considerably short of presenting a methodology for transforming health care providers into marketing organizations. This will be the task of a subsequent volume.

Contrary to some opinion, the U.S. health care industry is a vital, active enterprise, which has already undergone profound structural changes which will benefit both the patient and society. As society's needs change, major opportunities are being created for new forms of health care and new ways of meeting peoples' needs.

When combined with the increasing focus on economic competition, the structural changes already taking place will create major entrepreneurial opportunities in what has been, traditionally, a risk-averse industry. Physicians and hospital managers will face a changing strategic environment, one which will put the economic interests of the physician and the hospital into increased conflict. Changing economic opportunities will challenge hospitals and physicians to redefine the terms of their often troubled relationship, and seek mutual opportunities in an era of increasing scarcity of patients and income. The advent of scarcity, after decades of unimpeded economic growth and prosperity, will force both managers and professionals to rethink how they define their businesses, and how they relate to the patient, the ultimate consumer of health care.

The essence of a marketing approach to health care is that providers of health care, managers and professionals, will be compelled by increased competition to define and redefine their activities in terms of the needs of the patient and an increasingly resource-constrained society. In the best sense of the term, entrepreneurship requires an ability to understand people's needs and a willingness to devise new ways of meeting them. The price of a static definition of organizational or professional purpose in a changing world may be economic failure. In an economic competition there must be losers as well as winners. Those health care providers who understand the competitive framework within which they operate, and who are willing to redefine their business to meet peoples' changing needs, are likely to be the winners. To the extent that policymakers can liberate the entrepreneurial energy of health professionals and managers, the society may be the ultimate winner.

Acknowledgments

The ideas that gave rise to this book grew out of an administrative rather than an academic matrix. Many of the perspectives which helped shape those ideas came not from theorists but from practitioners of medicine or health management with whom I have been fortunate to work during my career at the University of Chicago. Many people took time to talk with me, or to read this manuscript in draft, and without their help I could not have written it. They should be absolved, however, from any responsibility for the ideas themselves.

Through extended conversations, several people helped me clarify issues that arose in their areas of particular expertise. Dr. Edward Newman of Michael Reese Hospital helped me understand more about the private practitioner and what he or she expects from the hospital. Dr. Thomas Frist, Jr. of Hospital Corporation of America helped define the emerging role of the hospital management firm in the health care industry. Dr. James Campbell of Rush Presbyterian-St. Lukes Hospital and Medical Center shared the perspective of an institution builder on how hospitals should relate to one another and to the physicians and patients they serve. John Shattuck of the Chicago-based Blue Cross Blue Shield and Karl Nygren of the law firm of Kirkland, Ellis discussed with me the uses and limits upon the power of health insurers to change the health care system. Fred Fink of Booz Allen Hamilton helped me explore the applicability of models of corporate strategy to health enterprises. George Caldwell of Lutheran General Hospital helped acquaint me with the objectives and techniques of hospital corporate restructuring. Robert Donnelly and his health care financing group at the First National Bank of Chicago helped me understand the capital manager's perspective on a changing industry.

Several other people read the manuscript in part and helped identify issues which needed clarification or rethinking. Clarence Teng of the Samaritan Health Service of Phoenix, Arizona critiqued the chapters on structural changes in the hospital industry. Michael Koetting of the Illinois Health Finance Authority and Sheila Mahtesian of the University of Chicago Medical Center's Social Services Department critiqued the chapter on aftercare. David Murdy, a student in the Pritzker School of Medicine, critiqued the chapter on health maintenance. Ann Zercher of the University of Chicago Medical Center's Nursing Department critiqued the chapter on the nursing shortage. Peter Snow of Booz Allen Hamilton read and critiqued the market analysis in the first half of the book, and offered suggestions on clarifying its presentation.

A smaller group of brave individuals read the whole manuscript and offered both organizational and substantive advice on its contents. Robert Vraciu of the Center for Health Studies at the Hospital Corporation of America, Odin Anderson of the University of Chicago Center for Health Administration Studies, Dr. Bruce Flashner, a physician with broad policy and managerial background who is the founding partner of The Flashner Medical Group, Richard Knapp, Director of the Department of Teaching Hospitals of the Association of American Medical Colleges and my father, Gerson Goldsmith, an attorney who was a commissioner of public welfare and of comprehensive health planning and former chairman of the Health Facilities Cost Review Commission of the State of Oregon, all made helpful suggestions which led to a clearer presentation of the issues.

Several people who work with me at the university made major contributions to the research upon which the book is based. They include Lynn Carter, Laurel Olson (now at the American Medical Association), Douglas Fair, and Mark Golberg. Their assistance in assembling background documentation from a wide variety of sources was invaluable. Patty Seymour not only researched several of the chapters but typed and assembled the manuscript, no mean feat given her administrative duties in running the office of health planning and health regulatory affairs of this Medical Center. She did an exceptional job in all of these things.

Two people made it possible to write this book by providing me the freedom to translate what I have learned as an administrator into this book. They are my colleague, David Bray, who is executive director of the University of Chicago Hospitals and Clinics, and my boss, Robert Uretz, who is dean of the University's Pritzker School of Medicine. As one of them put it one day, "Jeff, as long as we get our 50 hours a week from you, you can do anything you want." Other than for tolerating my researches, they are both to be held blameless for any opinions or policy implications of this book. They are my own, and do not represent the policy or views of the University of Chicago, a great university.

Jeff Goldsmith
University of Chicago Medical Center

Contents

Foreword   vii

Preface   xi

Acknowledgments   xvi

List of Figures   xxi

1. The market for health care: An overview   1
2. Ambulatory services   25
3. Aftercare   49
4. Health maintenance   77
5. Hospital strategy in a maturing market   97
6. Horizontal consolidation: The multi-hospital system   107
7. Vertical integration   135
8. Physician and the hospital   161
9. The crisis in nursing: Implications for the hospital   183
10. Conclusion   201

Appendix: What you need to know about your hospi-
   tal's competitive position   205
Bibliography   225
Index   235

LIST OF FIGURES

1–1 Selected components of the consumer price index, 1967–1979   8

1–2 Distribution of national health expenditures by type of expenditure   10

1–3 Total inpatient days in nonfederal short-term, and other special hospitals   15

1–4 Days of care per 1,000 population by selected age groups, 1965–1978   16

1–5 Competitive alternatives to hospital care   17

2–1 Annual percentage increase in physicians' average professional net incomes and average professional expenses, 1971–1979   28

2–2 Total inpatient days and surgical days: Short stay and specialty hospitals, 1968–1978   39

3–1 Relative growth of over 65, and over 75, and over 85 population   51

3–2 National health care expenditures by type and percent of total, calender years 1940–1979   52

3–3 Inpatient days by type   54

3–4 Nursing home revenues   56

3–5 Participating home health agencies, June 30, 1971–1980   67

4–1 Levels of satisfaction with various aspects of available health care service: Net difference between members and nonmembers   86

4–2 HMOs owned or managed by national firms   94

6–1 Total beds and units   109

6–2 Multihospital systems by type of ownership   110

6–3 Control and impact by type of system   111

6–4 Change in selected characteristics of 200 systems surveyed (1975 and 1979)   113

6–5 Contract management summary   115

7–1 Hospital feeder system, 1940   138

7–2 Type of visit in selected medical settings: Percent distribution of ambulatory physician visits   140

7–3 Hospital feeder system, 1960   140

7–4 Hospital feeder system, 1980   143

7–5 Corporate organization chart   156

8–1 Continuum of physician compensation arrangements   165

8–2 Comparative cost structure: Group practices and hospital outpatient clinics   176

9–1 Where are RNs working   188

9–2 How degrees affect your income   192

9–3 Which services pay best   193

A–1 Estimates of population required per health professional   210

A–2 Nonfederal physicians, civilian population, physician-population
ratios and rank by state, 1978   221
A–3 Ratio percent of projected supply to estimated requirements-
1990   222

1

The market for health care: An overview

Private industries and businesses which operate in free-market competition have developed a management discipline to guide their organizations' relationship to their customers. That discipline is called *marketing*. Though there has been a recent flurry of interest in marketing in the health care field, particularly for hospitals, the concept remains cloudy in the minds of many health professionals and managers. Marketing conjures up a complex of unsavory images, which include manipulation, promotional "hype," and high-pressure tactics. The prevailing popular image of marketing is anathema to professionals, whose own organizations until very recently forbade them to engage in it.

Yet it will become clear from the analysis which follows that health professionals and managers have already entered an era of heightened competition for patients and health resources. To approach this milieu without a competitive strategy will become increasingly foolhardy. As we will make clear below, marketing is a strategic activity, of which the highly visible promotional activities conventionally

1

viewed as synonymous with marketing are only a small part. Marketing is not a set of tactical maneuvers in which you engage only when you have encountered competitive difficulty. Rather, it is a management function which involves making sound strategic choices which shape the organization's role and competitive position in the health system.

THE MARKETING CONCEPT

Underlying modern corporate marketing management is what has come to be known as the "marketing concept," which first surfaced in business literature in the mid-1950s. Though many people played a role in its development, the key articulator of this concept was Peter Drucker. Drucker viewed marketing as central to any business. This centrality related to his view of the role of the customer:

> If we want to know what a business is we have to start with its *purpose*. And its purpose must lie outside of the business itself. In fact, it must lie in society since a business enterprise is an organ of society. There is only one valid definition of business purpose: To create a customer.[1]

In Drucker's view, the role of the organization in relation to the potential customer is active, not passive:

> Markets are not created by God, nature or economic forces but by businessmen. The want they satisfy may have been felt by the customer before he was offered the means of satisfying it. . . . But it was a theoretical want before; only when the action of businessmen makes it effective demand is there a customer, a market.[2]

Thus, a marketing orientation begins *outside* the organization, with the customer, current or potential. The marketing concept, as Drucker enunciated it, turns that customer's needs into an organizational mandate that involves all those activities—product development, pricing, promotion and distribution—that result in satisfying his needs. Thus, the marketing concept views the whole organization from the standpoint of its final result—delivery of customer satisfaction. To Drucker, a business which neglects the customer, that is, which fails to focus its attention on what the customer needs, is ultimately destined to fail.

In a famous *Harvard Business Review* article entitled "Marketing Myopia,"[3] Theodore Levitt extended the marketing concept by examining the history of businesses, indeed whole industries, which failed because they took the customer, and implictly, the market for their products, for granted. Levitt saw the definition of a firm's "business"—its purpose—not as static but as constantly changing as the society and its needs change.

Since organizations develop bureaucratic inertia, they mistakenly assume that the market for their product will not change and that the job of the organizations is to "produce" and "sell" the product. In a production-oriented business, the marketing task is to sell the firm's output. Selling is *not* marketing. Selling takes the product and demand for it for granted. Marketing realizes that the demand for any product is likely to change as the customer's needs change and that innovation is essential to keep pace with changing social needs. Levitt extended Drucker's core concept of the need to define one's business in terms of the customer into a mandate, even an imperative, for organization renewal.

Thus, a commitment to the concept of marketing implies a willingness to re-examine the purpose of the business more or less continually and to alter the organization and its products to respond to changing needs. Marketing-oriented organizations are continually evaluating their image, products, and philosophy in terms of the customer's needs and perceptions. Many of the nation's commercial success stories of the postwar era—Eastman Kodak, Polaroid, IBM, McDonalds, Procter and Gamble, Revlon—were preeminent marketing companies which put this concept of marketing into practice.

Philip Kotler of Northwestern University is generally credited with broadening the marketing concept to nonbusiness applications in a 1969 article in the *Journal of Marketing*.[4] He followed this article with the publication of a text, *Marketing for Nonprofit Organizations*, in 1975.[5] His generic definition of marketing covered activities in both the business and non-business sectors:

Marketing is the analysis, planning, implementation, and control of carefully formulated programs designed to bring about voluntary exchanges of values with target markets for the purpose of achieving organizational objectives. It relies heavily on designing the organization's offering in terms of the target markets' needs and desires, and on using effective pricing, communication and distribution to inform, motivate, and service the markets.[6]

For our purposes, however, we will define marketing in simpler terms: *Marketing is all those activities which involve creating, sustaining, and managing the demand for what an organization produces.* The key concepts here include defining an organization's "product" and conceptualizing the "demand" for it, which inevitably is generated by some groups or group outside the producing organization. The idea that organizations can *manage demand* is the most important part of the definition and is likely to be mildly counterintuitive both for health care professionals and managers.

THE APPLICABILITY OF THE MARKETING CONCEPT TO HEALTH CARE

The management tasks of any service organization, profit or nonprofit, are more complex than for a typical manufacturing enterprise. The "product" of most service enterprises is intangible. One cannot store, stack or count, or drop-ship "health" or "financial security." Thus, many of the marketing technologies of industry, particularly those which relate to logistics, laboratory research and development, and physical distribution, do not apply to most service industries. Further, because the product is intangible, it is difficult to measure productivity in the sense of definable, manageable relationship between input (labor and goods) and output (product). While it is inherently more difficult to manage service organizations for productivity, as will be seen later, it is eminently possible.

Because they tend to be dominated by professionals whose primary commitment is to their own professional practices, health care enterprises and their managers tend to be production-oriented. That is, they take the organization's current service offerings, and their quality, accessibility, and other important variables, for granted. To the extent that they engage in marketing activities, they tend to be oriented toward selling the product to a customer whose needs are, more often than not, defined in a self-serving way.

While this orientation is unlikely to be problematical in a sellers market, where providers of health care are in short supply, it may be disastrous in increasingly competitive markets. While the relationship of a physician to a patient may generate personal satisfaction, professional rewards flow from peers not from patients. Further, physicians may be specifically concerned if the hospital at which they practice mismanages their own patients and are more likely to judge a hospital by how well it serves *their* needs than by how well it serves their patients' needs. Unless directly threatened economically, individual physicians are likely to have no interest in whether their hospital's "market share" is slipping.

Health care is *not* a commodity; it is the most intimate personal service. The personal nature of the transaction between physician and patient, and the fact that most such relationships (except for family practice) involve the physician in seemingly isolated dyads (pairs), obscures the underlying similarities between patients. The similarities between one physician's practice and another's are likely as well to escape notice. Underlying this fragmentation are some common concerns, however.

Patients expect their physician to be reasonably accessible, and they expect to trust his or her medical judgment in managing their illnesses. They also have some concerns about the reasonableness of the fee, since they are likely to bear a greater portion of that cost than for other services. They expect some reasonable congruence of moral values and attitudes toward some forms of medical treatment (abortion, for example). They expect the relationship to be confidential. Indeed that confidentiality is often a precondition to effective diagnosis of any illness. Any of these expectations may be disappointed, of course, and may lead the patient to seek care elsewhere.

Thus from the patient's point of view, the physician's product is effective, sound, medical management, delivered with competence and concern. In general, physicians do relatively little actively to build their medical practices beyond trying to care competently for existing patients, relying on word-of-mouth and personal contacts to provide new patients. Because until recently physicians have operated in a seller's market, they have not had to concern themselves seriously with feedback from patients.

From a hospital's perspective, the core market is the physicians who practice on its medical staff. Though hospitals have relatively recently begun to dilute their risk by providing pathways into the hospital (emergency room, problem clinics, etc.) which do not require direct physician mediation, hospitals must rely on their medical staffs to bring in the vast majority of patients. The two mediating variables which govern hospital utilization are the vitality of the physician practices of medical staff members and the share of hospitalization of the physician's patients that she or he chooses to bring to the particular hospital. Thus, the true market for hospital services is the physician.

However, to serve the physician effectively, the hospital must do two things: meet the physician's needs for efficient service and support for his or her medical activity *and* meet the patient's needs for convenient, quality hospital care. For hospitals which have extensive referral practices, such as tertiary level teaching hospitals, the patient's family physician, who refers the patient to a specialist who manages the care in-house, must also be accommodated.

In the first instance, application of the marketing concept to the hospital requires a responsive relationship between hospital administration and the medical staff. However, the matrix relationship between hospital administration and medical staff (dual lines of authority which must act in an interdependent fashion), poses the problem of where to lodge the responsibility for looking beyond the hospital's current programs to define future organization. Since physicians control utilization, marketing cannot be exclusively an administrative activity. Because medical practices are isolated from one another, it is frequently difficult to get physicians to view the medical needs of the community as a whole. These factors inhibit the development of a marketing orientation in hospitals but do not excuse the failure to adopt it. When the hospital begins losing money it becomes easier to get everyone's attention. Unfortunately, by then it is often too late to solve the problem.

THE SPECIAL ROLE OF THE HOSPITAL

In order to understand the importance of a marketing orientation for health care providers, it is essential to understand the structure of the health care market. Because the largest single segment of that market is the hospital industry, exploring the demand for hospital services is the best place to begin.

The hospital is the institutional core of the nation's health care system. It is the focal point for the community's physicians, as well as a powerful social and political institution. The hospital is also the most capital-intensive (and capital-hungry) component of the health care system, a fact which will loom ever larger as the cost of capital continues to escalate. Originally, hospitals were charitable institutions, built in the best American tradition through acts of private philanthropy and, subsequently, through public works. These charitable origins account for the not-for-profit status of most of the nation's hospitals.

However, beginning in the 1930s with the founding of Blue Cross plans and accelerating in the 1960s with the enactment of Medicare and Medicaid, an increasing amount of health care and virtually all hospital care, became covered by some form of health insurance. Stimulated by the increasing breadth of coverage and fed by rising demand for health care as almost an entitlement, the hospital industry in the United States has grown into a major economic force.

Hospitals accounted for $85.3 billion in expenditures during 1979, fully 40 percent of the nation's total health care spending.[7] This amount will certainly exceed $100 billion in 1981. There were 6,988 hospitals in the United States during 1979, containing approximately 1,370,000 beds. Of this total, 5,923 hospitals were community hospitals, which accounted for 988,000 of the beds. On any given day, more than 1 million people awaken in a hospital bed.[8]

Given the enormous physical plant and volume of care, it is not surprising that hospitals are among the nation's largest institutional employers, with a work force of almost 3.8 million people[9] and an annual payroll of $41.5 billion. Among

FIGURE 1–1
Selected components of the consumer price index, 1967–1979
(all urban consumers)

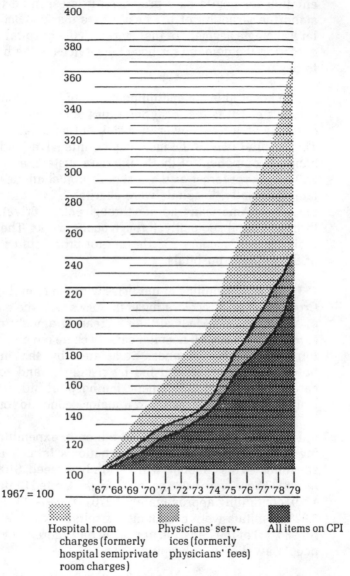

1967 = 100

Hospital room charges (formerly hospital semiprivate room charges)

Physicians' services (formerly physicians' fees)

All items on CPI

Source: Reprinted from Jeff Goldsmith, "The Health Care Market: Can Hospitals Survive?" *Harvard Business Review,* September–October, 1980. Data for 1967–77: *Handbook of Labor Statistics 1978* (Washington, D.C.: Bureau of Labor Statistics, U.S. Department of Labor); 1978–79 data: phone conversation, Bureau of Labor Statistics, July 1, 1980.

the people are almost 81,000 physicians, nurses, and other health care personnel in training.[10]

Through the major federal health care entitlement programs, Medicare and Medicaid, government has become the largest purchaser of hospital services. Almost 35 percent of the nation's hospital bill is paid for by the Medicare and Medicaid programs.[11] Government also exercises a major role as a direct provider of hospital care through the Veterans Administration hospital system, armed forces hospitals, state mental-hospital systems, and local public/general hospitals, though this role has been declining in recent years. Total government outlays for hospital care, for direct service, and through third-party payment, total $47.7 billion, or 56 percent of the total hospital bill in 1979.[12]

Because government pays so much of the nation's hospital bill, government budgets are sensitive to rising hospital costs. As can be seen from Figure 1–1, for most of the last 15 years hospital costs have risen much more rapidly than the rate of general inflation in the U.S. economy.

Since 1965 hospital spending increased from $13.9 billion to over $85 billion in 1979 (see Figure 1–2).[13] Hospital spending thus accounted for 42 percent of the total increase in health care spending since 1965. By 1979 hospital expenses accounted for 74 percent of total Medicare spending and 36 percent of Medicaid spending.[14] Hospitals have supplied the largest aggregate spending pressure on federal and state health care programs.

Since Medicare and Medicaid spending play a major role in federal and state budgets, hospital cost increases have become a political issue. They played a major role in precipitating financial crises in New York City and in the states of Massachusetts and Illinois during the 1974–75 recession. As a result, there has been an escalating effort at the federal, state, and local levels to contain hospital costs.

Efforts to secure direct federal cost controls on hospitals during the Carter administration were rebuffed by Congress. Thus, most federal efforts have focused on the so-called

FIGURE 1–2
Distribution of national health expenditures by type of expenditure

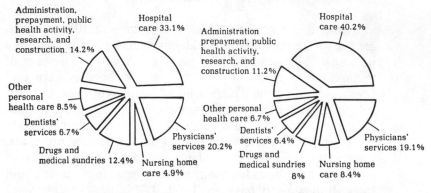

Calendar year 1965   Calendar year 1979

Type	1965 ($ millions)	1979 ($ millions)
Hospital care	13,885	85,342
Physicians' services	8,473	40,599
Administration, prepayment, public health activity, research and construction	5,993	23,649
Drugs and medical sundries	5,212	17,807
Other personal health care	3,550	16,975
Dentists' services	2,809	14,220
Nursing home care	2,072	13,607
Total	$41,994	$212,199

Source: Data and chart from Robert Gibson, "National Health Expenditures, 1979," *Health Care Financing Review*, Summer 1980, pp. 21–22.

Health Planning program, and most state efforts on public utility-style hospital rate review.

CONTROL OVER HOSPITAL-BED SUPPLY

Federal health policy during the post-World War II period has been characterized by a broad swing from active federal encouragement of expanded hospital-bed supply to active federal efforts to reduce supply. In 1946, with strong rural backing, Congress enacted the Hospital Survey and Construction Act, popularly known as the Hill-Burton Program. The purpose of the act was to help assess areas of hospital underservice in the country and to provide federal matching grants to construct new hospitals in areas where they were needed. From 1947 to 1971, the federal government committed $3.7 billion in federal funds, which generated a total investment of nearly $13 billion in health facilities through Hill-Burton. The program resulted in the construction of an additional 340,000 hospital beds, mostly in small towns and rural areas.

State Hill-Burton agencies were compelled by the act to assess the need for facilities in their areas in order to secure federal funding. During the early 1960s New York State went beyond Hill-Burton mandates and established the nation's first Certificate of Need program, which required hospitals to obtain prior approval from a state agency before proceeding with construction. As cost pressures mounted during the late 1960s and early 1970s (especially as a result of the recessions of 1969–70 and 1974–75, which sharply increased state Medicaid outlays for hospitals), more states enacted Certificate of Need laws, until by 1979, 46 states had such legislation.

During the late 1960s, federal policymakers began to view the fragmentation of the health care system as an increasing problem. Through the Partnership in Health Act of 1966 they created a network of voluntary state and local planning agencies to engage in comprehensive regional planning for health care. However, beyond the vague mandate to coordinate federal health resources in given areas, it was far from clear what these agencies intended to accomplish. Given this mandate, it surprised no one that they accomplished very little.

In 1974, facing growing concern over the growth in Medicaid and Medicare spending, Congress replaced the comprehensive health planning agencies with a new network of agencies which were given a clearer mandate to engage in planning and regulatory activities. Under the Health Planning and Resource Development Act of 1974, Congress established local health planning agencies called Health Systems Agencies and state health planning agencies, and a set of review functions mandated to "shrink the system." Guidelines issued under this act called for reduction of bed supply in the country to a level of four beds per 1,000 population and the achievement of a variety of more specific objectives.

Underlying the mandate to shrink the system was a theory that if hospital beds exist they will tend to be used. This theory is called the "Roemer effect," after the researchers who documented higher hospital use rates in high-supply areas. To the extent that hospital beds are *not* used, policymakers argued that the society would pay for allegedly high fixed costs of the unused beds. The result is a federal policy mandate which can be likened to compelling an overweight person to reduce weight by restricting the size of his clothing. Yet despite the best efforts of a newly created cadre of bureaucrats and self-anointed "health care consumers," hospital capacity continued to expand and hospital costs continued to increase. Congressional ardor for the program has cooled considerably, and the Reagan administration has proposed shrinking the health planning system as a fiscal move. There is no compelling (even circumstantial) evidence that the annual federal expenditures in excess of $150 million for each year of the program have returned commensurate benefits to the taxpayer. Fifteen years of experimentation with two versions of health planning have not produced either the coordination or the cost reductions sought.

In fact, by increasing the entry barriers for new hospital providers, regulatory efforts may have hardened the monopoly power of existing providers. Regulatory barriers to outside competitors have substantially strengthened the credit standing of existing providers by assuring bondholders that new competition is unlikely. While retailers who are successful in a given market area have absolutely no assurance that competitors will not set up shop across the street, Certificate of Need has virtually assured the successful hospital that new entrants will not steal their market. By enfranchising existing providers, regulation may have protected inefficient providers from better managed competitors.

RATE REGULATION

By the late 1960s states had begun to apply public utility regulation concepts to hospital care through the establishment of state-level rate review. More than two dozen states adopted rate-review mechanisms for hospitals during the 1970s. The results are at best inconclusive. Though one recent research effort has established that in six states where rate review was well established, expenses per admission rose less rapidly than the national average,[15] this study is clouded by the fact that several of these states, notably New York and Massachusetts, throttled back their Medicaid programs due to fiscal crises during the study period.

Alain C. Enthoven argues that the combination of industry efforts to alter the hospital care base, industry capture of regulators, and perverse incentives of cost control mechanisms may do little to influence hospital costs, let alone to increase hospital efficiency or productivity. As he says:

> The general history of economic regulation in our country does not support the presumption that regulation reduces costs to consumers. Indeed, the present moves to deregulate transportation are based on powerful evidence that regulation has raised costs.[16]

The burden of proof that extra-market mechanisms are effective in restraining hospital costs remains on those who advocate such approaches. The emerging consensus of health policymakers in Congress and elsewhere is that regulation has failed in other sectors of our economy and has yet to demonstrate significant results in the health care industry.

COMPETITION IN THE HEALTH CARE FIELD

Led by Enthoven and others, health care analysts have focused attention on encouraging competition as a means of increasing efficiency and reducing the rate of increase in health care costs. The existing third-party payment systems have insulated both the consumer and physician from the economic consequences of consuming health care.

However, even those who advocate these competitive approaches to restructuring the insurance system ignore the intense competition which does exist between providers of health care for patients and patient revenues. Much of this competition has focused on convenience to the consumer and physician and the quality and comprehensiveness of care available. However, competition between different modes of delivering health care is a force which many policymakers have ignored, because the trade-offs and competitive relationships between these modes are not clearly understood. Hospital managers and physicians are certainly aware

that they operate in a competitive milieu. Mediated by reimbursement policies that govern what insurers are willing to
pay for, this competition may, by reducing demand for the
most expensive modes of care, ultimately have a much more
profound effect on health care costs than regulatory approaches.

DEMAND FOR HOSPITAL SERVICES

As mentioned above, hospitals are the core institutional
provider of health care in the United States. Yet as hospital
costs continue to rise and press against the outer limits of
taxpayer and insurer willingness to pay for increases, hospitals will become increasingly vulnerable to competition from
less expensive and more convenient modes of rendering
health care, as well as to wholesale reductions in levels of
reimbursement from public health care programs. Much like
the urban department store, which faces major competition
from alternative retailing modes (drug store chains, discount
houses, direct mail, boutiques, and specialty shops), hospitals face competitive threats from alternative modes of
rendering health care, including health maintenance organizations (HMOs), ambulatory surgical centers, freestanding
urgent care centers, and ironically, their own medical staffs.
Many of the newer forms of care have in common the substitution of outpatient for inpatient care with both cost and
convenience benefits to the patients. Other forces, such as
the declining use of the hospital for long-term and chronic
care, and the growth of mechanisms such as HMOs. which
ration hospital care, has also reduced the demand for inpatient care. New forms of health care will reduce utilization
of the hospital's core service line of inpatient care in the
next few years, perhaps significantly.

It is impossible to document the extent of these trade-
offs completely. Though a Blue Cross study showed that Blue
Cross subscribers used 18.6 percent fewer inpatient days
of care and 137.6 percent more outpatient visits in 1978 than
they did in 1968, it is impossible to determine how much
of this shift was due to changing health status of enrollees
or change in the composition of those who are insured.[17]

The extent of economic trade-offs between different forms
of care can and will be accelerated by growing insurer efforts

FIGURE 1–3
Total inpatient days in nonfederal short-term, and other special hospitals

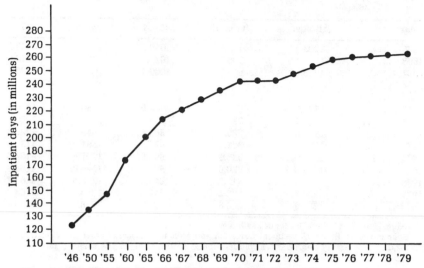

Note: Average daily census multiplied by 365 for selected categories.
Source: American Hospital Association, *Hospital Statistics* (Chicago: American Hospital Association, 1980) pp. 5–6.

to make more aggressive use of their medical purchasing power. The impact of this shift in utilization may be that the demand for inpatient hospital care will decline over the next 20 years, even given the projected increase in the elderly population.

Recent hospital utilization data bears out this contention. While community hospital inpatient days increased by 27.5 percent from 1965 to 1975, they have increased by only 2.9 percent in the five years from 1975 to 1979 (Figure 1–3). This is despite the growth in the number of elderly of approximately 2.5 million during the same period. Hospital outpatient utilization appears to have plateaued as well. Outpatient clinic visits increased by only 7.5 percent during this five year period but actually declined by 1 percent during the last two years of the period.[18]

Underlying this trend in aggregate hospital utilization is a decline in per capita hospital inpatient use during the same period (Figure 1–4). Average inpatient days consumed per

FIGURE 1–4
Days of care per 1,000 population by selected age groups, 1965–1978
(short-stay hospitals)

Year	All ages	Under 15	15–44	45–64	65+
1965	1203.4	408.6	1040.2	1710.9	3443.5
1966	1221.4	398.8	1025.3	1718.8	3712.0
1967	1238.9	410.9	1000.1	1634.6	4086.2
1968					
1969					
1970	1172.7	332.9	903.9	1550.0	4015.4
1971	1143.1	327.2	869.2	1535.0	3860.3
1972	1199.9	329.5	886.8	1642.7	4076.8
1973	1211.6	321.9	878.5	1661.0	4136.4
1974	1232.9	328.4	891.6	1701.8	4107.0
1975	1254.9	328.0	885.1	1748.9	4165.9
1976	1236.0	317.2	843.8	1716.8	4163.7
1977	1236.7	308.2	849.2	1688.3	4156.3
1978	1224.9	304.8	824.7	1638.7	4183.8

Note: Data for 1968 and 1969 not available.
Source: United States Department of Health and Human Services, Center for Vital Health Statistics, *Utilization of Short-Stay Hospitals—United States*, selected years, series 13.

1,000 U.S. citizens *peaked* during 1975 at approximately 1,255. This number has since declined by 2.4 percent. The typical American is consuming fewer hospital days now than five years earlier. Declines are even more abrupt for the two largest segments of the U.S. population, those under 15 and those between 15 and 44 years of age. Use rates for those under 15 declined by 7.1 percent and for the bracket containing the baby boom population, by 6.8 percent. Though use rates for the elderly seem to be holding firm, (despite the best efforts of the professional standards review organization [PSRO] program), hospital utilization has virtually plateaued in the aggregate for the U.S. population and has declined on a per capita basis in the last five years.

What has produced this development? There are three broad competitive forces (Figure 1–5) which affect the demand for inpatient hospital care and which will exert a major influence on hospital use patterns in the future. They are: the growth and diversification of ambulatory care, the growth of alternative delivery systems including HMOs, and the growth of aftercare for the chronically ill and the elderly. Growth in these alternative modes of rendering health care will reduce the demand for inpatient services in the future.

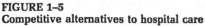

FIGURE 1–5
Competitive alternatives to hospital care

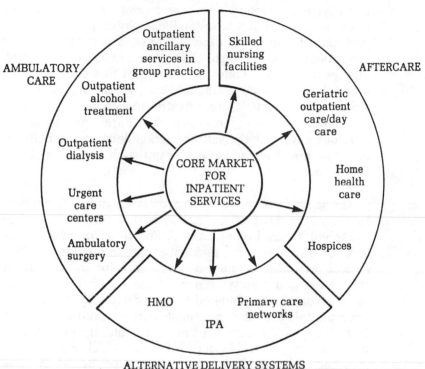

The first sector, *ambulatory care,* has both grown and diversified. Spurred by scientific advances and changing medical technology, much care that was rendered inside hospitals 20 years ago can now be rendered on an ambulatory basis. Advances in drug therapy for many mental disorders and development of community-based treatment helped empty out mental institutions. Development of drug therapy for tuberculosis shut down most of the large chronic disease hospitals during the postwar period. Many types of surgery can now be performed without hospitalizing the patient through "day surgery" or ambulatory surgical programs. Many types of emergency care, short of massive trauma, can be rendered outside the hospital in freestanding emergency facilities.

On top of these developments, physicians have developed more complex practice settings which permit them to perform many types of diagnostic work in their offices or group prac- tices, rather than in a hospital. Since physicians control the provision of ambulatory care, they have the ability to redirect the patient from the hospital to office settings they control, and recapture the economic rewards of this care from the hospital. For reasons related to the increasing supply of phy- sicians, the economic pressures on physicians to compete with the hospital will increase in the future. The trends and developments in the physician marketplace and in ambula- tory care are discussed at length in the chapter on ambula- tory care.

The second sector which represents a significant competi- tive threat to hospital utilization is that range of services to the elderly and chronically ill known as *aftercare*. This sector, which comprises residential care in nursing facilities as well as in-home and outpatient care for the elderly, is the most rapidly growing part of the health care system. Much medical care rendered to the elderly may not be most appropriately provided in an acute-care hospital setting. Fur- ther, much of the care needed by the elderly may not be medical care at all, but social service, which need not be provided by medical personnel. Federal policymakers have recognized this by encouraging rapid growth, first of nursing facilities and, subsequently, of home health care services over the last 15 years. Growth and development of this sector will be explored in the chapter on aftercare.

The third sector is comprised of the so-called *alternative delivery systems,* such as HMOs. More than 9 million Ameri- cans are now enrolled in some form of prepaid health plan.[19] Patterned after the successful Kaiser Permanente Medical Care Program of California, health maintenance organiza- tions contract with physicians, hospitals and other providers to render all the health care their members need. Health maintenance organizations charge a fixed fee, determined in advance, for meeting the health care needs of their mem- bers and serve as a prime contractor in arranging their care. The prepayment feature, and the fact that illness is a cost to the HMO rather than potential income to the provider, encourage HMOs to economize in the purchase of medical care. Since HMOs have a major economic incentive to reduce utilization of expensive hospital services and to substitute less costly forms of care if possible, they represent a competitive threat to hospitals. The growth of these systems will be explored in the chapter on alternative delivery systems.

The last 20 years have witnessed dramatic structural changes in the health care system in the United States. New forms of health care and new systems for providing that care have emerged, encouraged by growth in federal financing of health care but fueled by entrepreneurship, both small scale and large scale. There is intense competition within each of these sectors, as well as between hospitals and alternative modes of rendering health care. This competition will increase in the future.

THE ROLE OF MEDICAL PURCHASING POWER

Only about one third of the nation's health care expenditures, or $60 billion, were made directly by Americans in 1979.[20] The remaining two thirds of personal health expenditures were either generated by government grants and direct delivery by government agencies, or through private health insurance and government health care entitlement programs such as Medicaid and Medicare. The design of these reimbursement systems has generally accommodated itself to the central role of the physician by separating his reimbursement from that of the hospital, and by reimbursing the hospital for its costs incurred (more or less) as the physician has dictated. Beginning with professional standards review organizations, however, government and other third party payers have begun to encroach upon the physician's judgment to eliminate medically unnecessary hospital expenditures.

Up to this point, most insurers and payers of health care have attempted to achieve structural change and induce efficiencies in the purchase of care by fostering alternative modes of rendering health care through extension of health benefits to new types of services. Medicare and Medicaid sought to trade off lengthy hospital stays by creating lower cost extended care facility reimbursement, as well as reimbursement for in-home services. Recent amendments to Medicare and Medicaid laws liberalized reimbursement for ambulatory surgery conducted outside the hospital. Government and private payers have moved cautiously in fostering the growth of alternatives because it is nearly impossible to document the cost-saving trade-offs that may result.

There are signs, however, that the government and insurers may begin to take the alternative approach of being increasingly specific about what they will pay for and in what settings. Several state governments are experimenting with reimbursement of hospitals on the basis of diagnosis, rather than purchase of services on a per diem basis. While the initial intent of the so-called Diagnosis-based Reimbursement Group (DRG) system is to correct hospital per diem costs for the relative sickness (intensity) of the hospital's patients, DRG systems also provide the data base for deciding whether certain diagnoses will be reimbursed *at all* in certain settings. Purchase of hospital services on a diagnosis rather than per diem basis is expected by policymakers to encourage more rapid discharges and more efficient means of rendering care, because hospital costs will be covered only to a certain point, not ad libitum. This departure from cost-based reimbursement, which is blamed for much hospital cost inflation, could profoundly alter the ground rules under which medical care is rendered and accelerate the trading off of inpatient care against other forms of care.

At the same time, insurers are becoming less willing to pay carte blanche for whatever services may be provided to patients. Blue Cross, for example, has declined to reimburse hospitals for batteries of ancillary tests which are automatically rendered to the patient upon admission to the hospital. The California Medicaid program (MediCal) requires special documentation before it will reimburse inpatient stays associated with certain surgical procedures which can be done on an outpatient basis.

There are political limitations on the ability of government health programs to impinge seriously on the physician's discretion in rendering health care. It is unlikely that the government will be able to alter the fee-for-service reimbursement mode for physicians significantly. At the same time, the fiscal pressures created by public demand for tax relief and increased defense spending will inevitably force federal policymakers to re-examine the effectiveness with which they are purchasing health services for the vast populations of indigent and elderly served by its entitlement health programs. This pressure may result in increased efforts to purchase health care according to more precise definitions of medical needs. Alternatively, it may simply result in initiatives which reduce payment for care by government programs, forcing providers to economize or withdraw from servicing the populations. While the physician may be able to render care and derive income from alternatives, the hospital may be the net loser.

At the same time, private insurers are running out of margin in absorbing increasing hospital costs, and may begin applying increasingly stringent tests of necessity before paying for health care. Insurance policies are likely to become increasingly specific about what types of care will be rendered for what conditions. Increasing selectivity of health insurance benefits will accelerate trade-offs which already exist between more and less expensive modes of rendering health care. If these trade-offs are aggressively pursued, either through competitive brokering or through increasing specificity of insurance coverage, demand for the most expensive forms of health care delivered in hospitals could be reduced significantly.

THE SPECIAL ROLE OF THE ELDERLY

Though individuals over 65 constitute only about 10 percent of the U.S. population, they consume almost 30 percent of the nation's health resources. This population is expected to grow by almost 25 percent between now and the turn of the century. Many in the hospital industry believe that the growth in the elderly population will mean increasing demand for hospital services, since the elderly currently consume almost four times as much hospital care per capita as the national average.

However, there are two factors that may reduce the aggregate impact of the increasing elderly population on demand for hospital services. First, state and federal budgets are already seriously strained by the combined impact of the growth in elderly population and inflation. It is unlikely that the federal government will continue to be able to pay for four days of hospitalization per capita for the elderly, and will begin to force trade-offs with aftercare alternatives to hospitalization.

✓   The amendments to Medicare passed by Congress in the winter of 1980 move federal health policy in this direction. First, under certain circumstances, hospitals may be denied hospital-level reimbursement for services rendered to patients who are awaiting nursing home placement but do not need acute medical care. Smaller hospitals are encouraged to develop "swing beds" which can be converted from acute care to long-term care as needed. Second, the amendments liberalized home health care benefits under Medicare and began to loosen some nursing home reimbursement standards as well. While demand for health services for the elderly will undoubtedly increase, how much of this increase will be shared by hospitals remains to be seen.

The second factor which could blunt rising demand for hospital services is the changing health status of the elderly. In a recent article in the *New England Journal of Medicine,* Dr. James Fries contended that the increases in life expectancy during this century occurred not because of a lengthening of the absolute span of life as much as because of a reduction of premature deaths due to infant mortality, infectious disease, and other acute illness.[21] Fries argues that medical advances and healthier lifestyles (e.g. more exercise, reduced smoking, proper diet, and weight control) will reduce the period of morbidity prior to death by postponing the onset of chronic illness. Fries argues that the mean age at death is biologically fixed. Fries goes on to say:

> The social consequences of this phenomenon will be profound. Death and disability, occurring later, become increasingly unavoidable. The incremental cost of marginal medical benefit inevitably rises. Intervention in the patient without organ reserve will be recognized as futile.[22]

While it is difficult to imagine patients and physicians abandoning curative approaches to prolonging life, what Fries suggests is that there may be growing acceptance of "palliative" care which accommodates to the inevitability of death and that peoples' attitudes toward incurring the expense of acute care will change.

It is impossible to quantify the impact which healthier lifestyles will have on the consumption of health services. But it is becoming increasingly apparent that everyone can have an enormous impact on his or her own health status by proper exercise, diet, and the avoidance of known health hazards such as smoking.* Ultimately, the individual may have more influence on the demand for hospital services than the physician and the insurer together. The healthier the population, the less likely it is to consume as much hospital care as the current elderly population. The corresponding demand of tomorrow's elderly for hospital care will be proportionately diminished.

CONCLUSION

The health care industry in the United States is undergoing profound structural changes which will alter the role the hospital and the physician play in rendering medical care. As this structure broadens and diversifies, alternatives to acute care hospitalization will become increasingly attractive economically. The more rapidly hospital costs escalate, the more rapidly these trade-offs will be forced by health insurers. Just as the rising price of oil increases the economic viability of substitute fuels, the rising price of hospital care will encourage growth of ambulatory services, alternative delivery systems, and aftercare for the nation's elderly. As costs increase, competitive pressures within the hospital industry will intensify to the point where many hospitals, perhaps hundreds, may be forced to close, and as many as several thousand others may be absorbed by large hospital management firms. Entrepreneurial opportunities will abound in many areas outside the hospital as well.

These developments can only benefit the patient, because it will present him or her with an array of cost-effective, convenient alternatives for receiving health care. As competition for patients increases, both physicians and hospitals,

---

* These factors may already account for the declining per capita consumption of hospital services among the 15 to 44 age group discussed above.

as well as other providers of health care, will be increasingly interested in meeting the patient's needs. The patient will no longer be what one famous health services analyst called the "breathing brick" of the health care system. Consumer sovereignty will be a watchword of the competitive health care system.

NOTES

1. Peter F. Drucker, *The Practice of Management* (New York: Harper & Row, 1954), p. 37.
2. Ibid.
3. Theodore Levitt, "Marketing Myopia," *Harvard Business Review,* September–October 1975.
4. Philip Kotler and Sidney J. Levy, "Broadening the Concept of Marketing," *Journal of Marketing* 33 (January 1969).
5. Philip Kotler, *Marketing for Nonprofit Organizations* (Englewood Cliffs, N.J.: Prentice-Hall, 1975).
6. Ibid.
7. Robert Gibson, "National Health Care Expenditures: 1979," *Health Care Financing Review,* Summer 1980, p. 17.
8. American Hospital Association, *Guide to the Health Care Field, 1980* (Chicago: American Hospital Association, 1980), p. 4.
9. United States Department of Health and Human Services, Public Health Services, Office of Health Research, Statistics and Technology, *Health United States 1980* (Washington, D.C.: U.S. Government Printing Office, 1980).
10. American Hospital Association, *Guide to the Health Care Field, 1980,* p. 4.
11. Gibson, "Health Care Expenditures," p. 29.
12. Ibid.
13. Ibid., p. 32.
14. Ibid., p. 29.
15. Brian Biles, Carl J. Schramm, and J. Graham Atkinson, "Hospital Cost Inflation Under State Rate Setting Programs," *New England Journal of Medicine* 303, no. 12 (September 18, 1980): 664–67.
16. Alain C. Enthoven, *Health Plan* (Reading, Mass.: Addison-Wesley Publishing, 1980).
17. Blue Cross and Blue Shield Associations, "Blue Cross Plans Experience Sharp 10-Year Decline in Hospital Utilization Rate," press release, January 18, 1980.
18. American Hospital Association, *Hospital Panel Survey 1980* (Chicago: American Hospital Association, 1980).
19. "July 1980 Survey Results: HMO Enrollment and Utilization in the U.S." (Excelsior, Minn.: *Interstudy,* July 1980).
20. Gibson, "Health Care Expenditures," p. 29.
21. James F. Fries, "Aging, Natural Death, and the Compression of Morbidity," *New England Journal of Medicine,* July 17, 1980, pp. 130–35.
22. Ibid.

2

Ambulatory services

To the extent that anyone "controls" the health care system, it is the physician. Because of prestige and political power, the physician has escaped most direct regulation and has preserved a good measure of freedom to organize and conduct a practice as he or she sees fit. There is, however, no freedom from pressures of the market for health services. Today the physician faces considerable pressure both from expanding numbers of colleagues and from inflation. How the physician adapts to these market pressures will have a major bearing on the future organization of his or her services, and on the future of the hospital as well. In this chapter, we explore the diversification of the ambulatory services sector which the physician controls and the implication of economic competition on the structure of a practice.

MEDICAL PRACTICE—THE LAST FRONTIER

The practicing physician is one of the last surviving independent entrepreneurs on the American scene. Even more than other professionals, physicians seem to be infused with a powerful spirit of "don't tread on me." As we will discuss below, while the number of physicians in group practice is growing, over 60 percent of the 239,000 physicians in private office practice as late as 1976 were solo practitioners.[1] As a physician writing in the late 1960s put it:

> It was a need for freedom that made me choose solo practice . . . solo decisionmaking is at the heart of good medical practice and . . . a doctor's freedom to decide is to some extent compromised when he becomes part of an organization.[2]

Since physicians are entrusted with the management of people's health and can be held both legally and morally responsible for the loss of life, there are powerful reasons why physicians want to control as many as possible of the factors which govern whether they succeed. Professionals in general, but physicians in particular, are perfectionists and become accustomed to the unquestioned exercise of authority in their practice.

This exercise of power has economic consequences. An estimated 71 percent of the nonfederal physicians engaged in patient care in the United States are compensated through the fee-for-service system,[3] a hallmark of independent physician practice. The combination of largely unchallenged freedom to direct the practice of medicine with the piecework method of compensation has attracted severe criticism from some economists. This criticism has given rise to an image of the physician as "economic man" who abuses professional power to increase income by prescribing medically unnecessary treatment for patients.

Some of these critics have extended the argument to its logical conclusion—that physicians will generate enough demand for their services to permit them to reach a hypothetical "target income."[4] If competition from other physicians (e.g., in areas of high physician density) reduces the volume of patient visits, physicians will simply increase their fees to produce the same income level. Uwe Reinhardt, one of the most sophisticated (and wittiest) of these critics, believes that since each new physician will necessarily generate between $250,000 and $500,000 in health care expenditures each year, restricting physician supply and compelling them to increase their productivity is the most effective way to restrain health care costs over the long run.

The debate over the merits of reimbursing physicians by methods other than fee-for-service, such as the capitation methods used by health maintenance organizations (HMOs), is likely to continue for some time. But the caricature of the physician as an omnipotent income maximizer fails on at least two counts. First, it fails to take into account the intense professional pride which most physicians bring to their practice and the nature of the satisfactions they derive from it. Frank Sloan, a perceptive observer of physician practice, has commented that

> neoclassical theory provides only the most general guide. . . . It was not designed to explain the behavior of trained professionals seeking more out of work than financial security at minimal levels of effort.[5]

Furthermore, the caricature bears only minimal relationship to what most of us know of our own physicians and their colleagues. Besides being vicious and demeaning, however, it does not reflect accurately the economic realities.

Economist critics argue that physicians have sufficient control over utilization to generate revenues so that they can set their income levels at will. If this is so, this theory does not account for certain recent developments in physicians' income and activity. One could reasonably assume that physicians would have used that power to hold themselves harmless from the recent inflationary surge. The facts do not bear out this contention.

Two surveys of physician income trends established that physician net incomes declined during the 1970s on the average. In 1979, analysis of the American Medical Association's annual survey of its membership established that, during the 10 years 1970 through 1979, gains in physician net incomes (pretax) fell considerably short of keeping up with inflation. During this period physician practice costs increased at an annual percentage rate of 8.3 percent, while *gross* professional income, which reflects fee levels charged for physician services, increased by only 6.7 percent. Physician net in-

FIGURE 2-1
Annual percentage increase in physicians' average professional net incomes and
average professional expenses, 1971–1979

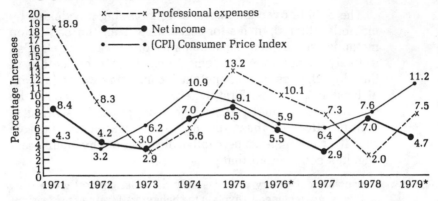

* = Expense and Income data for 1976 and 1979 projected by physician respondents.

Source: Periodic Survey of Physicians, 1972–1979, Center for Health Services Research and
Development (Chicago: American Medical Association). Consumer price index data from *Handbook of Labor Statistics, 1978* (Washington, D.C.: Bureau of Labor Statistics, U.S. Department
of Labor) for 1971–77 Data; For 1978–79 Data, telephone conversation with Bureau of Labor Statistics, July 1, 1980.

comes increased at an annual average of 5.7 percent, compared to an annual rate of increase in consumer prices of
7.2 percent. According to the AMA data, the slippage accelerated in the last three years of the decade. In 1979, consumer
prices increased by 11.3 percent while physician net income
grew by 4.7 percent.[6]

As can be seen from Figure 2–1, physicians net income
lost ground to inflation in every year after 1972. While data
are not available to explain precisely why practice costs
rose so sharply in 1971 and in the 1975–77 periods, one can
speculate that they reflect sharp, nonincremental increases
in the cost of malpractice insurance, and labor cost catch-
up following two periods of high inflation. It is strongly suspected that the brunt of this cost and income pressure has
been borne by the new entrants into the physician marketplace, and that these averages mask sharp gradations of
activity and income between generations of physicians.

In a survey of physicians conducted by *Medical Economics* for the five-year period from 1975 through 1979, a similar

finding was established. For all specialties, the five-year loss in the purchasing power of net income was 4 percent, comparing 1979 median incomes to 1974 dollar value. Of the various specialty groups, only orthopedic surgeons and internists were able to stay ahead of inflation. By contrast, pediatricians lost about 9 percent, general surgeons about 10 percent, and obstetricians and gynecologists almost 12 percent. Furthermore, only 43 percent of the physicians surveyed expected their practice earnings in 1980 to be higher than in 1979, while 13 percent actually expected them to be lower (in actual, rather than constant, dollars).[7]

Several things must be said to put these findings in perspective. No data was gathered by either survey on trends in physician *net worth,* which may have increased more rapidly than inflation, particularly as "bracket creep" and changes in the tax laws encouraged physicians to shelter more of their income. Also, it must be noted that even given the diminution of purchasing power, average physician salaries are still substantially higher than for most of the rest of us. The AMA average net income for all specialties was $68,999 in 1979,[8] while the *Medical Economics* average net income was $76,720.[9] Physicians continue to be our wealthiest occupational group by a wide margin. But they are not immune to the economic realities of inflation. Their economic powers, while considerable, have not enabled them to escape inflation's pressures.

Even more significant, however, is evidence of declining physician activity levels. Data on the median number of visits per physician week, showed a decline of 13 percent from 1974 to 1980 for all specialty groups. Some specialty groups showed even steeper declines over longer periods of time. General practitioners surveyed showed an approximate decline of 22 percent from 1972 to 1980 in median weekly visits, while general surgeons showed a 21 percent decline over 10 years.[10] Independent confirmation of this trend is available from federal health survey data, which showed a nearly 4 percent decline in the number of reported physician visits between 1975 to 1978. The per capita visit rate for persons of both sexes dropped from 5.1 to 4.8 visits during the same period.[11] Many physicians appear to be working at less than full capacity and not necessarily by choice.

Several factors may be at work in producing income and activity trends. Economic conditions may have reduced discretionary consumption of physician services. They may also have prevented physicians from collecting income from increasingly hard-pressed patients even though they continue to increase their fees. It is suspected that patients may be less willing to pay physician fees than other expenses because they perceive that the physician is wealthy and can afford to lose the income. Professional fee receivables undoubtedly contributed to the growing gap between gross billings and net income. Unfortunately, data to substantiate this suspicion are not readily available.

But other factors of greater long-term significance may be at work on the physician supply side. The growing number of medical practitioners may have begun to affect physician professional activity and incomes. During the period of the AMA survey, the number of physicians in the United States increased by over 30 percent. The outlook for physician supply suggests that competitive pressures will increase rather than diminish in the future. These pressures will reshape the practice of medicine, creating both challenges and opportunities for physicians.

OUTLOOK FOR PHYSICIAN SUPPLY

In 1976, David Mathews, secretary of what was then the Department of Health, Education, and Welfare, created a body called the Graduate Medical Education National Advisory Committee (GMENAC) to advise him on the nation's future health manpower needs, and on the appropriate federal policies for meeting those needs. This study, the most comprehensive analysis of medical manpower yet conducted, not only mapped past growth in the number of physicians in various specialty areas but, using a sophisticated model of demographic, epidemiological, scientific and technological trends, projected needs in the various medical specialties for the year 1990.

The final report of this body estimated that by 1990 the nation will have approximately 536,000 physicians, 33 percent more than in 1978 and 79 percent more than in 1970. This total represents approximately 70,000 more than the GMENAC study estimated will be needed in 1990. The projected surplus will double to 145,000 during the following ten years.[12] The goodness of fit between projected supply and projected needs varies considerably according to specialty, with persistent shortages predicted in psychiatry, emergency medicine, and preventitive medicine. Some surgical and medical sub-specialties such as neurosurgery, endocrinology, and pulmonary medicine are projected to produce nearly double the number of specialists needed by the year 1990. Tables showing these projections are in the Appendix.

The report also predicts little progress in resolving the serious geographical maldistribution of physicians. For example, New York State has nearly two and a half times as many practicing physicians per 100,000 people as Alabama. Statewide physician-to-population ratio data may also be found in the Appendix. These data mask substantial disparities within states between suburban and inner city areas. For example, the large inner city area surrounding the University of Chicago had only 773 physicians in practice for a population of almost 1.2 million during 1976, a ratio of physician-to-population coverage reflecting only about half of the statewide average for Illinois.

Physicians prefer to practice in areas where it is desirable to live, where cultural and recreational opportunities exist commensurate with their income expectation. This predisposition is strengthened by the reimbursement policies for the Medicaid program, which is the dominant payer for physician services in many inner city and less prosperous rural areas. In Illinois, for example, the Medicaid reimbursement rate for a basic physician's office visit in 1980 was $10.50, much less than half the prevailing level of charges in the area. These reimbursement policies have aggravated physician supply problems in areas where there are large numbers of poor people.

Perhaps unwittingly, Congress worsened the supply outlook for many inner city and rural areas in 1976 when, in response to organized medical pressure, it tightened restrictions on the entry into the United States of foreign-trained physicians. The GMENAC report recommended further restriction of so-called foreign medical graduate (FMG) entry into the United States as one step toward reducing the impending surplus of physicians. Municipal hospitals, which deliver large amounts of care to the inner city poor, as well as state mental hospitals and hospitals in some rural and depressed suburban areas, are differentially dependent on FMGs, who frequently fill gaps created by practice preferences of American trained physicians.

How these patterns of geographical distribution change in response to further growth in physician supply remains to be seen. There is some evidence from a recent Rand Corporation study that medical specialists are moving into rural areas and small towns in increasing numbers.[13] It is reasonable to speculate that physician density in highly desirable areas (southern California, for example) will continue to increase until the market signals to potential newcomers that it is saturated. Research on the behavior of local or regional physicians markets in these areas should be conducted, both because little is known about them and because these market conditions presage conditions in the rest of the country.

Increasing competition between physicians seems likely to continue to retard the growth in physician net incomes and compel physicians to re-examine the structure within which they practice. New entrants into the physician market, and there are now more than 17,000 of them annually, will be compelled by competitive conditions to develop new and more effective methods of delivering primary physician services. These pressures are likely to produce structural changes in the physician-controlled sphere of ambulatory care as profound as those taking place within the hospital industry.

STRUCTURAL CHANGE IN AMBULATORY PRACTICE

In economic terms, a physician's practice is a small business. For solo practitioners, such enterprises may gross as little as $50,000 to $100,000 a year, while large group practices might gross as much as several million annually. These solo and group practices accounted for most of the $40 billion in direct physician economic activity in 1979 and, indirectly, for a significant portion of the $85 billion in hospital expenditures in the country during the same period.[14] While there has been some growth in new forms of physician practice in recent years and increased interdependence among physicians due to increasing specialization, the modal unit of production of physicians services has changed little in the last hundred years. Some of the reasons for this were discussed above and include the physician's desire to control his or her own destiny. However, market forces may create financial trade-offs for this "freedom" which new entrants into the physician market may be either unwilling or unable to make. Some of the likely changes in the structure of physician practice are discussed below.

INCORPORATION

For many years, organized medicine has opposed the "corporate" practice of medicine.* Many states enacted statutes to forbid lay control over medical practice, on the grounds that it would compromise the quality of patient care. As medical practice has emerged as a major economic force, attitudes toward the physician's role in corporate organization has moderated somewhat. By 1980 virtually every state has a professional incorporation statute which permits some form of corporate structure for professional medical practice, mandating explicit physician control over the corporation. Though the percentage of physicians who participate in incorporated practices rose sharply during the 1970s, only about half of practicing physicians in the United States participated in incorporated medical practices as of mid-1979.[15] The tax and other advantages to incorporation yield much greater returns to physician income than unincorporated practice does. In 1979 incorporated physicians grossed 64 percent more than their unincorporated colleagues and netted 42 percent more. The spread for solo practitioners was even more dramatic, with incorporated solo practitioners grossing 72 percent more than solo unincorporated practitioners and netting 48 percent more.[16,]† These data are somewhat misleading since the ability to incorporate is conditioned upon generating sufficient after-tax income to be able to support the physician's financial obligations and lifestyle.

---

* A 1949 Report to the American Medical Association House of Delegates most clearly enunciated this policy: ". . . it is illegal . . . and unethical for any lay corporation to practice medicine and to furnish medical services for a professional fee which shall be so divided as to produce a profit for a lay employer, either individual or institutional (hospitals and medical schools)."

† The net figures for incorporated physicians represent pre-income tax earnings including bonuses and tax deductible retirement contributions.

The true advantages to incorporated practice lie in the tax sheltering of retirement benefits and the fringe benefit advantages of incorporation. Most self-employed individuals are permitted to invest $7,500 or 15 percent of their gross income, whichever is less, in Keogh retirement plans and reduce their taxable income by such investments. Under incorporation, physicians are able to deduct substantially larger percentages of their income for participation in corporate profit sharing and pension programs. The resulting takedown of gross income produces tax advantages many times larger than Keogh plan provisions.

In addition, incorporation permits physicians to deduct personal health and, in group settings, group life insurance premiums as a corporate expense, eliminating the need to pay for these essential fringe benefits with expensive after tax dollars. Under certain circumstances, physicians may even loan themselves funds from their own retirement assets set aside. These tax provisions permit the incorporated physician to shelter large amounts of current income from taxes and to build large equity bases not permitted the unincorporated colleague.

There are two chief reasons why physicians do not incorporate. First, they may not be taking home enough income to be able to afford to take advantage of the tax benefits of incorporation (e.g., to make the retirement plan contributions). Second, incorporation requires time, legal assistance, paperwork, and additional recordkeeping that some physicians are simply not willing to invest. They may also involve sharing benefit plans with employees, which is an expensive proposition. It seems clear, however, that additional financial pressures may compel more physicians to modernize the organizational setting within which they practice. It is strongly suspected that the proportion of physicians practicing in incorporated settings will continue to grow.

GROUP PRACTICE

For years, medical economists have inveighed against physician resistance to practicing in groups, arguing that the sharing of facilities and support costs and the continuity of physician relationships benefited the patient both economically and medically. As few as fifteen years ago only 11 percent of the physicians in practice in the United States practiced in groups.[17] In 1980 an AMA study established that approximately 88,000 physicians practice in groups, more than double the number in 1969. However, despite this growth, only about 26 percent of practicing physicians are part of groups.[18,*] Though the attitude toward group practice among recent or impending graduates of medical school may be moderating, the long-standing professional attitude toward group practice has been unremittingly hostile.

The first public expression of organized medical sentiment toward group practice was a 1920 policy statement on the possible infractions of ethical standards which might be inherent in group practice.[19] In 1927, when the University of Chicago opened its Hospitals and Clinics, the salaried group practice organization of its medical faculty provoked angry reaction from the Chicago medical community. The university's staffing plans were regarded as the "corporate practice of medicine" by practitioners in the community. In response to this reaction, the university was compelled to conclude an agreement with the Chicago Medical Society to see only as many patients as were absolutely essential for teaching and research purposes and not to charge professional fees for the services of its faculty.

Though economists such as Reinhardt have advocated consolidation of solo physician practices into large-scale groups, recent research has undercut the claim that large group practices produce significant economies. A number of these studies, reported by Richard Ernst, found that "the optimal or most productive scale of practice occurs at the small-group level."[20] Frank A. Sloan put the most efficient scale of group practice at about six physicians, quite far indeed from the large "medical corporations" envisioned by some critics.[21]

---

* The American Medical Association Council on Medical Services defines group practice as "the application of medical services by three or more physicians formally organized to provide medical care, consultation, diagnosis and/or treatment through the joint use of equipment and personnel, and with income from medical practice distributed in accordance with methods previously determined by members of this group." Two-person practice is usually termed *partnership*.

The income advantages to group practice for the physician appear to correlate with group size as well. According to AMA survey data for 1977, physician net income was highest among physicians who practiced in five- to seven-person groups, and the next highest for those practicing in three-person groups. The average net income for solo practitioners was 6.4 percent below the average for all physicians and 21 percent below that of the physicians in five- to seven-person groups.[22] Thus, while there is evidence that physicians in solo practice sacrifice considerable net income for the autonomy which solo practice provides, there is little evidence that large scale groups serve the physician's economic interests much more effectively.

While there appear to be some income advantages to physicians in group practices, it is not clear that these advantages are produced by the return on physicians' services alone. Some theorists have suggested that group practice is a vertically integrated form of "production" with two outputs—physicians' services and ancillary (laboratory and radiology) services.[23] The returns from the physician component of practice alone are not impressive, and according to R. M. Bailey actually decrease slightly as the group grows larger.[24]

However, those specialists (internists, general practitioners, orthopedic surgeons), which are heavily dependent on ancillary services such as X-ray and clinical laboratories, can generate significant fractions of their total practice income from ancillary services and capture an increasing amount of the economic rewards for their practice. Ancillary services are highly profitable in an office setting, because work is usually done by relatively low-paid technicians and the physicians themselves interpret the results rather than using expensive radiologists or pathologists. There are financial incentives for many practitioners to integrate ancillary production into the group setting. Ancillary profits are a significant incentive for the formation of groups, one which is likely to become more powerful as market pressures reduce the profitability of the physicians' services component of what a practice produces.

Thus just as we will see later in the case of hospitals, market pressures in the physician sector appear to create incentives to develop incorporated, vertically integrated structures for delivery of physician care. In their respective efforts to maximize physician income and market position, however, physicians and hospitals may be on a collision course. That is, as physicians develop more sophisticated forms of corporate organization, and begin to deliver (and hence control) a wider range of medical services, physicians will be increasing competitive threats to the hospitals in which they practice.

NEW FORMS OF AMBULATORY CARE

A principal thesis of this book is that economic pressures and market opportunities will compel physicians to offer a fuller range of medical services in settings they control. A variety of new forms of delivery of health care by physicians, as well as more sophisticated structures like vertically integrated group practice, present hospital managers with the possibility of significant losses of admissions, patient days, and (profitable) ancillary services volume. How hospital managers cope with this long standing but increasing competitive pressure may determine the long-run viability of their organizations.

Hospital diagnostic activity

A significant percentage of the inpatient admissions to the hospital are for diagnostic workups. Until comparatively recently, hospitals have offered the only convenient setting for the conduct of diagnostic tests, principally because of hospitals' near monopoly on diagnostic technology and because the logistics of working up a patient outside the hospital were too complex and inconvenient for the patient. With the growth of multispecialty practice, and the development of the hospital-independent ancillary services in these groups and in physicians' office buildings, this balance of technology and convenience may be changing. Furthermore, income sharing arrangements which permit the patient's primary physician to capture some of the financial return from those services which accrue to a hospital-based practitioner if the patient is admitted to the hospital, may create financial incentives to work the patient up outside the hospital.

In a Massachusetts study of hospital utilization patterns, Odin Anderson found that approximately 14 percent of hospital admissions in a large sample were for diagnostic purposes. When he probed the extent of physician discretion in these admissions, he found that only 45 percent of the procedures which necessitated admission were "impossible except in the hospital." Another 32 percent were considered "extremely difficult except in the hospital." Thus, almost one quarter of the admissions were "discretionary" in the sense that it was either possible or equally convenient to perform them outside the hospital. With advances in medical technology and in the concentration of medical practices over the last 20 years, it is strongly suspected that this percentage has increased. The combination of increasing extra-hospital logistical capability and economic incentives may significantly reduce the primary physician's rate of diagnostic admissions to hospitals in the future. The loss of hospital ancillary activity may, in turn, undermine the economic viability of the hospital by shrinking ancillary profits which are used, through cross-subsidization, to support such unprofitable activities as hospital-based ambulatory care.

Ambulatory surgery

Probably the most significant potential impact of the physician's increasing economic independence from the hospital is on a hospital's surgical utilization. Surgical utilization is the core of a hospital's inpatient volume. As can be seen from Figure 2–2, surgical utilization represented approximately 43 percent of the total community hospital inpatient days in 1978. From 1970–78, growth in inpatient surgical utilization accounted for 87 percent of the increase in hospital inpatient days.

In light of this important role of surgery in overall hospital utilization, the growth of freestanding ambulatory surgical (or "day surgery") programs poses a significant threat to hospital surgical programs. As much as 40 percent of all surgical procedures can be performed on an outpatient basis,[25] without either pre- or postoperative hospitalization. These procedures are concentrated in such "primary care" surgical specialties as otolaryngology, urology, and ophthalmology, as well as some more inpatient oriented specialties such as plastic surgery. The result may be a savings (to the patient and insurer) and loss (to the hospital) of from one to three days of hospitalization per procedure.

FIGURE 2–2
Total inpatient days and surgical days: short stay and specialty hospitals, 1968–1978

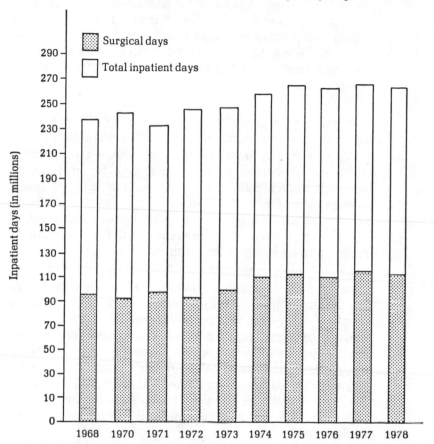

Source: Data obtained from National Center for Health Statistics, U.S. Department of Health and Human Services; and total inpatient data from American Hospital Association, *Hospital Statistics* (Chicago, 1980).

Though national data on the prevalence of ambulatory surgery is not available as of this writing, data has been obtained on one very active market—Phoenix, Arizona, with a metropolitan population exceeding 1.5 million. According to data assembled by the Central Arizona Health Systems Agency, nearly 28 percent of all surgical procedures performed in the region in 1979 were done on an ambulatory basis.[26] More than one third of the ambulatory surgical procedures were done in freestanding facilities. The Central Arizona HSA set an objective of having 40 percent of all surgery done on an outpatient basis by 1984, which appears to be an ambitious objective given past growth rates. Phoenix was among the first markets to embrace ambulatory surgery, as was similarly over-doctored Los Angeles. Physician supply in both these areas presages conditions in many parts of the rest of the country, suggesting that physician market pressures may have a good deal of influence on the growth of this type of surgery.

Ambulatory surgery offers a number of advantages to the patient, including minimized lost work or recreational time and the opportunity to be with friends or family during recovery. Instead of being admitted to the hospital for any required diagnostic work, patients are usually worked up in or through the physician's office. They will arrive at the surgicenter in the morning for their operation, spend the day recuperating from surgery in the facility, frequently with friends or family present, and go home in the evening.

Acceptance of ambulatory surgery will be accelerated by the liberalization of insurance benefits and by the growing acceptance of the concept by physicians and patients. Until relatively recently, federal health programs have favored hospital-based ambulatory surgery programs over freestanding programs in their reimbursement formulae. However, Medicare and Medicaid amendments in the fall of 1980 liberalized reimbursement policies for freestanding ambulatory surgical facilities, increasing financial incentives for their development.

Growth in ambulatory surgery may also be accelerated by the increasing reluctance of insurers to reimburse hospitals for inpatient stays associated with surgical procedures which can be performed on an outpatient basis (unless evidence is presented of complicating factors which require patient monitoring or full-scale inpatient surgery). Such developments will not necessarily damage the practice incomes of surgeons who have access to ambulatory surgical facilities (either hospital based or freestanding), but they could impede access to surgical services for those patients whose physicians do not have such access. The California Medicaid program (MediCal) will reimburse for many inpatient surgical procedures only if the physician documents either the lack of outpatient facilities for such surgery or the medical necessity of inpatient care associated with it. This demonstration must be made in advance of the surgery if it is to be reimbursed. This reimbursement practice is likely to spread to other states and other payers.

Many hospitals do have the option to develop their own "day surgery" programs, and for the stronger hospitals it may be an excellent strategy to pursue. However, movement in the hospital to day surgery can reduce its inpatient utilization unless the lost admissions can be replaced from other sources. In some cases, however, institutions may not have a choice. For example, Good Samaritan Hospital of Phoenix, was compelled by installation of a freestanding ambulatory surgical program in a physician office building across the street to create its own captive ambulatory surgical program.

One possible barrier to rapid development of freestanding programs may be the thinness of the malpractice coverage provided surgeons for nonhospital surgical practice. The hospital's malpractice insurance provides a convenient umbrella sheltering surgeons from potentially ruinous medical malpractice liability. The hospital's quality-assurance activities, required by federally mandated accreditation standards, provide malpractice insurers a rationale for more reasonable surgical coverage if procedures are performed in the hospital. Freestanding surgical practice does present greater exposure to the surgeon, though analysis of claims experience over several years may establish that the types of procedures performed on an ambulatory basis do not result in greater risk. This may, in turn, result in a softening of malpractice rates for freestanding surgical practice.

Hospital managers have reason to be concerned about the impact of freestanding ambulatory surgery on their operations, since surgery is another major profit center in most hospitals. The ability of hospital medical staffs to separate a significant portion of their surgical activity from the hospital poses a major threat to its overall inpatient activity. Hospitals which develop their own programs need not lose "facility" charges or ancillary volume but may be faced with empty beds.

Like the freestanding emergency facilities discussed below, freestanding ambulatory surgical facilities are eminently adaptable to franchise operation. Facilities plans, staffing, and financial systems are all amenable to standardization. It is not unreasonable to speculate that some of the corporate organizations moving swiftly into the health care market could develop "turn key" ambulatory surgical facilities which could be constructed and put quickly into operation in regional or national markets. Hospital management firms are more likely to build such programs into their base hospitals than to put up freestanding facilities, though the potential for damaging *competing* hospitals' surgical volume through strategically placed freestanding facilities may not be lost on some of these firms as local market conditions tighten. The key constraint on franchise expansion may be recruitment and retention of quality physicians to staff them.

Urgent care centers—freestanding emergency facilities

Hospi al emergency rooms are major contributors to inpatient utilization of the hospital. From 15 to 30 percent of all hospital admissions may come through the emergency room. In many urban areas emergency rooms have become the beneficiaries of many visits from patients who are not acutely ill but who have no physician or other means of getting care. Thus in many underserved areas 60 percent or more of the visits to the emergency room may be nonemergency cases. So not only is the emergency room an important source of inpatient admissions; it has become the health care system's current answer to the patient's need for episodic, nonscheduled health care.

Both for reasons of high cost and the "softness" of ER patient volume diagnostically, hospital emergency rooms are vulnerable to substitution of innovative methods of delivering episodic care. Such an innovation appeared on the horizon in the middle 1970s in the form of the urgent care center, or freestanding emergency facility. According to a study conducted for the Robert Wood Johnson Foundation, there were approximately 55 in existence in the United States in late 1978.[27] It is believed that many times that number are now in operation, though reliable estimates are not available.

These facilities can provide most of the services of a hospital-based emergency room except for full scale surgery (since they lack the capability of administering general anesthesia). However, they are capable of performing minor surgery, setting broken bones and applying casts, or stabilizing a stroke patient, as well as dealing with nonacute medical problems. Most facilities have their own laboratory and radiology facilities, though some contract these services out if rapid turnaround on tests at a reasonable cost is available nearby.

A network of such facilities has been developed in the Chicago area by a former health partner of Arthur Young and Company, Dr. Bruce Flashner. The name of the facilities, Doctors Emergency Officenter, cogently expresses the hybrid nature of the service. They operate 16 hours a day on a no-appointment basis. The first three facilities reached the breakeven level of patient visits within six months of their opening, in different northwest suburban Chicago locations.

Dr. Flashner experienced hostility from anxious physicians practicing near his facilities until it became clear that he did not intend to build an on-going practice through the centers. Patients are returned to their family physicians for continuing care or referred to specialists needed for complex conditions. In addition to a single physician per shift, a center employs three allied health personnel per shift who are cross-trained to handle billing, laboratory and radiology work, as well as to handle problems in patient flow through the facility. Dr. Flashner was able to avoid capital outlays in two of his facilities by leasing both facility and equipment. The capital costs of the leases were less than $100,000 per facility.

The facility is a cross between a private physician's office and an emergency room. It is a competitive threat to both. Such facilities bridge the gap between the frequently impersonal emergency room, where the patient may endure a lengthy wait, and the private physician's office, where the patient may wait days or weeks for an appointment. Competition from urgent care centers may force private physicians to allocate some appointment time to accommodate walk-in visits by their patients and to make afternoon and evening service available which is more convenient to patients with inflexible work schedules or other commitments.

Urgent care centers are a threat to hospitals because they deprive the hospital of control over the decision to admit a patient from the emergency room. Physicians in freestanding facilities have absolutely no incentive to hospitalize a patient, while the triage threshhold which admits a patient through a hospital-based emergency room may move up or down depending on the hospital's occupancy rate. Though no research has been done on the question, it is reasonable to speculate that the ratio of outpatient visits per inpatient admission may be much higher in a freestanding facility than in a hospital-based emergency room.

Nevertheless, hospitals anxious to increase their occupancy may offer physicians in urgent care centers preferential admitting privileges for patients referred for hospitalization. Because many hospitals rely on physician on-call lists to provide coverage for patients admitted through hospital emergency rooms, preferential access to referrals from freestanding facilities may mean, in practice, that a patient admitted through a freestanding facility can get admitted to the hospital more quickly than if he or she were admitted through the hospital's own emergency room.

As with ambulatory surgical programs, hospitals do have the option of developing satellite urgent care centers, which gives them control over patient flow even though emergency care is delivered offsite. An example of this strategy is the establishment of a captive freestanding emergency facility in the far eastern suburbs of Phoenix by the Samaritan Health Service. The facility feeds the easternmost network hospital in the Samaritan system for those emergency cases requiring hospitalization. It was established in a rapidly growing area to provide Samaritan a medical presence that could form the nucleus of another hospital if population growth continues at the current pace. Captive facilities provide hospitals control over the geographic origins of their patients and a relatively low cost method of entering new or developing markets.

Freestanding dialysis centers

Kidney dialysis originated as an extremely costly procedure for treating kidney failure that could be conducted only in an inpatient hospital setting. With expanded government funding for treatment of end-stage renal disease provided under Medicare in 1972, and as a result of significant technological advances, most dialysis can now be performed on an outpatient basis.

As dialysis became available to more individuals needing it, outpatient dialysis services developed in freestanding settings. About 280 freestanding proprietary and nonprofit facilities treated about 47 percent of all dialysis patients in 1979. A single, investor-owned firm, National Medical Care, operates 40 percent of these facilities.[28] Hospital-based outpatient dialysis programs compete with freestanding proprietary and nonprofit organizations for dialysis patients. Hospitals are at a competitive disadvantage because the Medicare cost allocation principles allocate full hospital overheads to outpatient dialysis treatment, making it much more expensive than care in freestanding units. The number of hospital-based dialysis programs dropped 7 percent, from 680 facilities in 1977 to 635 in 1979.

Competition is likely to increase as a result of federal regulations promulgated in late 1980 which subjected hospital-based outpatient dialysis rates to a prospective payment system, which may cause deficits in many hospital-based programs and encourage them to close. The Reagan administration's apparent intention to abolish the higher hospital-based outpatient dialysis reimbursement rate in favor of a consolidated single rate for hospital-based and freestanding centers may spell the end of hospital-based chronic dialysis programs.

Freestanding dialysis centers can affect a particular, highly specialized market for inpatient hospital services in an important way. Specifically, there are powerful economic incentives for freestanding dialysis centers *not* to refer patients to tertiary hospitals for kidney transplants. The obvious reason is that a successful transplant obviates the need for further dialysis, removing the referred patient from the orbit of the freestanding agency. Thus the growth and potential dominance of the freestanding facilities in the dialysis market could help dry up demand for transplant surgery, further affecting a hospital's surgical volume in another profitable area.

THE PHYSICIAN AND THE HOSPITAL

All the developments discussed above have a common consequence. By developing new forms of ambulatory care, many of which offset or reduce the need for hospital inpatient care, physicians represent an increasing economic threat to the hospitals at which they practice. The incentives to develop new corporate structures and new forms of ambulatory care, under physician control, will increase as economic pressures from physician competition encourage physicians to capture more of the financial rewards of patient care and share less of them with the hospital. Since the decision to hospitalize a patient rests with the *physician,* the economic balance of power between the physician and the hospital manager, always a sensitive one, is likely to tip in the direction of physicians (even given their increased numbers). And as hospital costs continue to escalate, insurers may come to realize that private physician care is one of the few remaining bargains in the health care market.

Because physician office-based care is not cost reimbursed, and because overhead is lower, physicians are able to compete effectively on price in precisely those areas which are hospital profit centers—particularly radiology, clinical pathology, and surgery. Further, since there is a direct connection between physicians' activity and their income, there are powerful entrepreneurial incentives both to reduce costs and seek more business. These incentives lead to substitution of technicians for expensive medical specialists in ancillary areas as well as to referral relationships between physicians within the same medical peer groups. Because the physician is largely unregulated, he or she can move much more quickly than the hospital to maximize opportunities.

Physician entrepreneurship presents an uncomfortable long-term dilemma for the hospital administrator. Insurance plans and health maintenance organizations shopping for bargains may increasingly bypass the hospital in seeking certain types of health care. This may strip the hospital of its current profit centers, leaving it a loose collection of unprofitable operations. Besides creating powerful incentives to develop new lines of business for the hospital, these developments will require rethinking the relationship of the physician to the hospital. Some thoughts about this relationship and the strategic choices facing both administrators and physicians will be found in Chapter 8, Physician and the Hospital.

NOTES

1. Frank A. Sloan, Jerry Cromwell, and Janet B. Mitchell, *Private Physicians and Public Programs* (Lexington, Mass.: Lexington Books, 1978) p. 46.

2. Anne Rankin Mahoney, "Factors Affecting Physicians' Choice of Group or Independent Practice," *Inquiry*, June 1973, p. 10.

3. Jon R. Gabel and Michael Redisch, "Alternative Physician Payment Methods: Incentives, Efficiency, and National Health Insurance," *Milbank Memorial Fund Quarterly/Health and Society* 57, no. 1 (1979): 39.

4. Uwe E. Reinhardt, *Physician Productivity and the Demand for Health Manpower* (Cambridge, Mass.: Ballinger Publishing, 1975), p. 11.

5. Sloan, Cromwell, and Mitchell, *Private Physicians*, p. 23.

6. Gerald Glandon and Roberta Shapiro, eds., *Trends in Physicians' Incomes, Expenses and Fees 1970–79, Profile of Medical Practice, 1980* (Chicago: American Medical Association, Center for Health Services Research and Development), p. 49.

7. "Earnings Survey," *Medical Economics*, September 15, 1980, pp. 120–21.

8. Glandon and Shapiro, *Trends in Physicians' Incomes*, p. 49.

9. "Earnings Survey," pp. 120–21.

10. Arthur Owens, "Doctor Surplus: Where Things Stand Now," *Medical Economics*, September 29, 1980, p. 63.

11. "Current Estimates from the Health Interview Study—United States 1976–1978," *Vital and Health Statistics*, Series 10, no. 115 (March 1977:29; no. 130 (November 1979).

12. Report of the Graduate Medical Education National Advisory Committee to the Secretary, Department of Health and Human Services, Volume 1, *Summary Report*, September 1980, p. 3.

13. W. B. Schwartz, J. P. Newhouse, B. W. Bennett, and A. P. Williams, *The Changing Geographic Distribution of Board-Certified Physicians* (Santa Monica, Calif.: Rand Corporation, 1980), pp. 4–7.

14. Robert Gibson, "National Health Expenditures, 1979," *Health Care Financing Review*, Summer 1980, p. 17.

15. Owens, "Doctor Surplus," p. 63.

16. Ibid.

17. Mahoney, "Factors Affecting Physicians' Choice," p. 9.

18. "Medical Group Practice in the U.S., 1980," Center for Health Services Research and Development, American Medical Association, *Research Notes* 4, no. 2 (Spring 1981).

19. Mahoney, "Factors Affecting Physicians' Choice," p. 9.
20. Richard Ernst, "Ancillary Production and the Size of Physicians' Practice," *Inquiry,* December 1976, p. 371.
21. Sloan, Cromwell, and Mitchell, *Private Physicians,* p. 81.
22. Glandon and Shapiro, *Trends in Physicians' Incomes,* p. 26.
23. R. M. Bailey, "Economies of Scale and Medical Practice," in *Empirical Studies in Health Economics,* ed. Herbert Klarman (Baltimore: Johns Hopkins Press, 1970), p. 269.
24. Ibid.
25. James E. Davis and Don E. Detmer, "The Ambulatory Surgical Unit," *Annals of Surgery,* June 1972.
26. Central Arizona Health Systems Agency, "Ambulatory Surgery Criteria and Standards," July 9, 1980.
27. "Preliminary Survey of Freestanding Emergency Centers" (Silver Springs, Md.: Orkand Corp., February 1979).
28. "Dialysis Reimbursement Squeeze Spurs New Management Services," *Modern Healthcare,* August 1980, p. 80.

3

Aftercare

The second major sector which is likely to offset significantly the use of inpatient hospital services is health and social services for posthospital and chronic disease care of the aged. This sector, which encompasses a range of residential, outpatient, and in-home services, is the most rapidly growing part of the health care system, and it is as intensely competitive as the hospital sector. Though the conceptual focus of this book has been the impact of changing patterns of health care delivery on the market for hospital services, the market for aftercare services is the focus of an equally lively debate regarding the economic and human merits of alternative approaches to meeting the needs of the elderly.

Those who believe that Medicare resolved the problem of caring for the nation's elderly will be disabused rapidly of this notion by examining the evolution of aftercare services under Medicare. While the enactment of Medicare provided comprehensive coverage for treatment of acute illness among the elderly, it left a legacy of confusion and fragmentation in dealing with chronic illness and medical and social problems which accompany aging. As Anne Somers commented:

> Medicare's obvious deficits with respect to long term care and the chronically ill are not the result of sloppy legislation or poor administration. The program simply was not designed with chronic illness in mind. We now know that this is *the* major unmet health need of older people, but we are less sure how to correct the situation.[1]

In this chapter, we examine the growing demand for health and social services to the elderly and some of the competitive implications of various strategies for meeting their needs for hospitals and other health care providers.

HEALTH CARE AND THE ELDERLY POPULATION

In marketing parlance, the elderly are the "heavy half" of the health care market. Though the nations' elderly amounted to only 10.9 percent of the population in 1978, they consumed nearly *one third* (29.4 percent) of the nation's health resources.[2] Per capita hospital expenditures for the elderly were $869 in 1978, more than double the $370 per capita spent on persons aged 19 to 64, and eight times the expenditures for people aged 18 and under. The elderly have a per capita physician's office visit rate of 6.3 per year, 50 percent greater than for age groups under age 55. They also account for 86 percent of the nation's nursing home expenditures.

Within the elderly population, the concentration of health service expenditures increases as a person nears death. Over 32 percent of all Medicare expenditures are made in the last year of life for those persons over 85 years of age.[3] While persons over 85 accounted for only about 9 percent of the over 65 population in 1978, they consumed six times the amount of hospital days per capita as persons under 65 and 50 percent more than all persons over 65.[4] Furthermore, this population of very elderly persons accounted for 35 percent of all nursing home days of care.[5]

In light of impending population growth among elderly groups, their current rate of consumption of health services poses a major fiscal and human problem for the U.S. health care system (see Figure 3-1). The number of Americans over 65 years of age has increased from 4 million in 1900 to 24.5

FIGURE 3-1

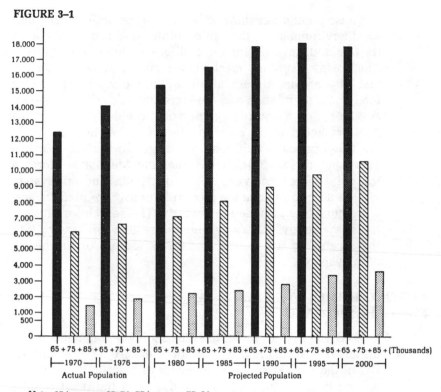

Note: 65+ means 65–74; 75+ means 75–84.
Source: *Health: United States 1978,* Washington: U.S. Department of Health and Human Services, p. 148.

million in 1980 and will more than double again, to an estimated 55 million persons, over the next 50 years. The elderly population is currently increasing at 500,000 persons per year.[6]

Within this group, the population aged 75 and over is expected to increase even more rapidly, reflecting the fruits of economic prosperity, advances in medical science, and the consequent improvement in health status of U.S. citizens. Those persons over 75 constitute 38 percent of the elderly population at present and those over 85, 9 percent. Those proportions within the elderly population are expected to increase to 45 and 12 percent respectively, by the end of the century. By the time the baby boom generation reaches the 75 plus threshhold, it will constitute more than half of the elderly population.

These population shifts will reshape the political and cultural environment in the United States and profoundly alter its tax and government expenditure policies and options. The social insurance mechanisms put in place during the last 40 years are already straining the federal budget under the impact of inflation and the increasing elderly population. As the ratio of working age persons to elderly declines, as it is projected to do dramatically over the next 40 years, the fiscal pressure will compel changes in the social insurance system for the elderly, including Medicare. More to the point of our analysis, it is unlikely that the tax system will be able to finance the mix and intensity of medical services currently provided the elderly. The search for alternatives is already underway and the results will restructure the incentives for growth in various sectors of the health care system.

NURSING HOMES—THE CORE MARKET FOR CHRONIC CARE

Over the last 30 years, the nursing home has become the principal institutional setting for the care of the elderly. Given the sharp rise in the numbers of elderly, it is not surprising that the nursing home industry is the most rapidly growing part of the health care system. As can be seen from Figure 3–2, nursing home expenditures in the United States grew from $187 million in 1950 to $17.8 billion in 1979. Since 1965 the share of the nation's health care outlays consumed by nursing home care has almost doubled, from 4.9 to 8.4 percent. During the 1970s nursing home expenditures grew at 19.6 percent annual rate, compared to a 12.5 percent rate for hospital expenditures.[7] The number of nursing home beds in the United States increased from 568,500 in 1963 to more

FIGURE 3–2
National health care expenditures by types and percent of total, calendar years 1940–1979 ($ millions)

	1940		1950		1965		1979	
Physician Services ..	$ 973	24.4%	$2,747	21.7%	$ 8,473	20.2%	$40,599	19.1%
Hospitals...........	$1,011	25.4%	$3,851	30.4%	$13,885	33.1%	$85,342	40.2%
Nursing Home Care	$ 33	0.8%	$ 187	1.5%	$ 2,072	4.9%	$17,807	8.4%

Source: Robert Gibson, "National Health Expenditures, 1979," *Health Care Financing Review* 2, no. 1 (Summer 1980), pp. 21, 22.

than 1.4 million in 1979. In 1978 nursing homes generated 452.8 million days of care, 74 percent more than all the nation's community hospitals for the same year.[8]

And yet, despite this substantial growth, only about 4 percent of the nation's elderly are presently in nursing homes, though several times this percentage of the elderly will use nursing homes at some point in their lives. Studies of the economics and market for nursing home care suggest that the recent explosive growth in capacity has not been sufficient to meet *current* demand, let alone the demand likely to be generated by the rapidly growing elderly population.

As Burton Dunlop has pointed out in his excellent analysis of nursing home demand, the growth in nursing home care is part of a larger trend toward increased institutionalization of the elderly. In part this trend reflects the growing economic power of the elderly, supported by social security and Medicare. But it also reflects among younger people a declining willingness or interest in supporting their parents in their own households, given the availability of alternatives. While it is true that the primary predictor of nursing home demand is the size of the older segment of the elderly population, population increases alone do not account for the extent of the growth in institutionalization.[9] While the number of elderly rose by 21 percent between 1960 to 1970, the number of institutionalized elderly rose by almost triple that rate— 58 percent. And the number of elderly in nursing homes *doubled* during the same decade, accounting for the vast majority of growth in institutionalization during the decade.[10]

The growth in nursing home care occurred at the expense of alternative settings for long-term or chronic care. Figure 3–3 shows postwar trends in the utilization of several of these alternative modes of care for the long-term patient. By 1979 days of care in mental institutions (nonfederal) had declined by more than 72 percent from the 1955 peak. Care in long-term general hospitals declined by over 46 percent during the same period. Care in the nation's veterans hospitals has declined by one third from the 1960 peak.

A number of factors governed the extent of the trade-off between nursing home care and these alternative modes of

FIGURE 3–3
Inpatient days by type

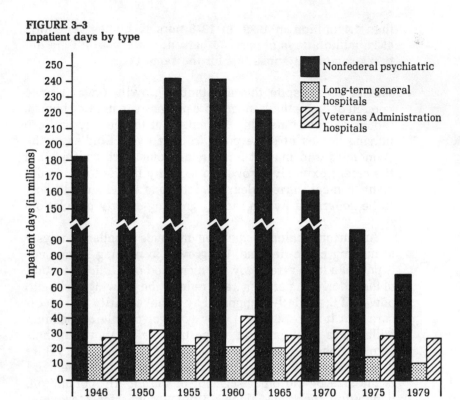

Note: Average daily census multiplied by 365 for selected years.
   Source: American Hospital Association, *Guide to the Health Care Field* (Chicago: American Hospital Association, 1980). Veterans Administration Hospitals, *Annual Report* (Washington, D.C.: U.S. Government Printing Office, selected years).

rendering long-term or chronic care. The movement toward "deinstitutionalization" of the elderly in mental institutions for example, reflected a number of convergent influences. They included advances in drug therapy, changing medical attitudes toward the appropriate treatment of senility, aggressive development of community based treatment programs, and changing fiscal incentives for state governments, principally as a result of the advent of Medicaid. William Pollak has estimated that 25 percent of the growth in nursing homes utilization between 1960 and 1970 can be attributed to diversion to nursing homes of patients either in or destined for mental hospitals.[11]

In the case of community hospitals, an increasing focus upon acute care led to a deemphasis on long-term care. In the last 25 years there has been a substantial shifting of demand for long-term care of the impaired elderly from hospitals to nursing homes. Dunlop observed:

> Until relatively recently, hospitals were often used to care for impaired and usually indigent elderly on a long-term basis, especially if they required any amount of nursing care. Some hospitals reserved special wings for long-term care, but this seems a largely post World War II development. Use was especially heavy for public charges in county hospitals. By the beginning of the study period (1960–1970), however, specialization of hospitals for acute care (with all its implications for facility prestige and rapidly rising costs) was nearly complete. This created increasing pressure to provide for the chronically ill or functionally impaired in specialized long-term care settings, principally nursing homes.[12]

As will be seen below in our discussion of Medicare and Medicaid impact on long-term care demand, one of the policy thrusts of Medicare was to encourage transfer of individuals recuperating from illnesses from hospitals to extended care facilities (ECFs). The impact of these shifts in hospital policy and insurance systems can be seen in the declining length of hospital stay during this same period of explosive nursing home growth. The length of stay in the nation's nonfederal short-term hospitals declined from 9.1 days in 1946 to 7.6 days in 1979, while the length of stay in public hospitals (nonfederal) declined even more dramatically, from 11.4 days to 7.4 days during the same period.[13]

Dunlop speculates that there was also some substitution of nursing home care for certain types of group care, including sheltered care and homes for the aged, as well as for residential living in unlicensed boarding homes, houses, and related facilities. The extent of this substitution is extremely difficult to document, though Dunlop pointed to a decline in the number of institutionalized elderly living in what the U.S. Census Bureau calls "group quarters"—from 40.5 percent in 1940 to only 12.3 percent in 1970. Dunlop points out, however, that much of this decline could also be attributed to the increased economic viability of independent living under social security.[14]

Medicaid and Medicare influence on the nursing home market

The impact of these two federal health care entitlement programs on nursing home demand is poorly understood by those outside the long-term care field. Few people realize, for example, that Medicare, the nation's entitlement health program for the elderly, finances only a minuscule portion of the nation's nursing home services (only about 3 percent in 1979), while Medicaid, the nation's entitlement program for the categorically needy, finances almost *half* of these services (Figure 3–4). In 1978 only 8.6 million days of nursing home care were covered under Medicare, 56 percent fewer than in 1968.[15]

There is virtually no private insurance coverage for nursing home services at the present time. In 1979, private insurance accounted for less than 1 percent of nursing home expenditures. The balance of financing for nursing home care is from the "self-pay" patient, as can be seen from Figure 3–4. When asked why there is no private insurance market for long-term care, industry experts point out that it simply has never been needed since it is so easy to enroll patients in the Medicaid program. The principal technique is to transfer the assets of the elderly to children or other relatives. Since financial resources of the children of the elderly are not considered in determining the elderly person's eligibility for Medicaid, the elderly will generally "spend down" remaining resources and become covered by Medicaid. Given the rapidly deteriorating outlook for Medicaid funding, the Medicaid role as the residual insurance mechanism for long-term care seems to be ripe for re-examination. Private insurance for supplemental nursing home coverage, and ultimately for the full cost of care, will come to be demanded by the nursing home industry and by consumers threatened with

FIGURE 3–4
Nursing home revenues, 1965 and 1979 ($ in millions)

	1965	Percent of total	1979	Percent of total
Total nursing home care	2,072	—	17,807	—
Consumers-direct (self-pay)	1,337	64.5	7,481	42.0
Private insurance	2	0.1	117	0.7
Other private programs	21	1.0	107	0.6
Medicare	—	—	373	2.1
Medicaid	—	—	8,796	49.4
Other government programs	711	34.3	934	5.3

Source: Robert Gibson, "National Health Expenditures: 1979," *Health Care Financing Review,* Summer 1980, pp. 29, 32.

diminished access to long-term care as Medicaid funding is curtailed.

The relative roles of Medicare and Medicaid in nursing home financing can be explained by reviewing the legislative history of these programs. The drafters of the Medicare legislation viewed the nursing home as a lower cost extension of the hospital for recuperation of the elderly patient. The thrust of the Medicare Extended Care Facility (ECF) program was thus to link Medicare funding of long-term care benefits to particular hospitalizations. Specifically, the legislation mandated a minimum three-day hospital stay prior to admission to a long-term care facility, certification of the medical need for admission by the patient's physician, and that the admission to the nursing facility take place no more than 14 days after discharge from the hospital. Coverage was limited to 100 days of long-term care per illness, with copayment by the patient after 20 days, presumably to encourage patients not to use the full 100 days.

During 1969, in an apparent response to the increased program costs of nursing home care under Medicare, the Department of Health and Human Services tightened eligibility standards by limiting care only to those individuals who had "rehabilitative" potential—excluding many of the chronically ill as well as the preterminally and terminally ill. The 1969 regulations also tightened the definition of services for which the program would pay, as well as the costs which it would reimburse as part of "reasonable cost" of care. These redefinitions led to retroactive denials of reimbursement for Medicare services already rendered, infuriating the nursing home industry and triggering massive provider defections from the program.

The result of restricting nursing home reimbursement under Medicare was to push the elderly into the Medicaid program, where costs were shared with the various state governments participating in the program. Thus the federal government avoided growing nursing home costs by shifting them onto state governments. Because Medicaid definitions of covered services were much broader than those of Medicare, many of the elderly who met income eligibility criteria for Medicaid became eligible for Medicaid coverage of their nursing home benefits.

As Dunlop points out, however, enactment of Medicaid did not result in large new populations becoming eligible for government-financed long-term care. The primary reason for this is that preceding programs under social security—the Old Age Assistance and Aid to the Aged Blind and Disabled Programs—already covered nursing home care. These programs, and related state-funded medical assistance programs, accounted for 34.4 percent of nursing home revenues in 1965, the year prior to implementation of Medicaid. According to Dunlop, "except in a very few states, the adoption of Medicaid seems to have had very little effect on the relative access of the population to nursing home care and hence on demand through the raising of income eligibility levels."[16] Rather, population growth and shifting patterns of demand for services, combined with more generous reimbursement, helped accelerate growth in the nursing home bed complement and population.

However, Medicare and Medicaid appeared to have a major impact on two key features of the nursing home—quality and the supply of beds. With respect to quality, the federal government began to require compliance with life safety and staffing standards as a condition of participation in the program. This, in turn, led to stricter state licensing laws for nursing homes and resulted in a dramatic upgrading in the quality of nursing home facilities. Dunlop illustrated the difference between pre- and post-Medicare/Medicaid periods as follows:

> In 1964, the typical nursing home was an older, wooden-frame two- or three-story converted house, containing perhaps forty beds, owned and operated by a husband and wife, with an LPN supervising staff activities during the day shift. Today, the Life Safety Code with its expensive provisions and the information and reporting requirements for participation in federal funding programs—principally Medicaid—has produced typically a single-story, fire-resistive facility of sixty beds frequently owned by a corporation or partnership of investors and often managed by a salaried nursing home administrator. It houses a larger proportion of sicker patients and employs RNs and/or LPNs supervising staff functions on all shifts.[17]

Of course, these standards also led to large increases in the unit costs of care (that is, beyond inflation) and is believed to have encouraged the entry of investor-owned firms into the nursing home management field.

On the reimbursement side, the introduction of the two programs established the legitimacy of cost-related reimbursement, which was the basis for Medicare reimbursement. For Medicaid, states were encouraged to move away from a flat, state-wide rate set independent of particular facility costs toward a facility-dependent rate. In most cases, this was open-ended "cost reimbursement," with a maximum level specified. Of course, the maxima became the equivalent of a fixed rate as facility costs moved upward rapidly toward them. In general, the implementation of Medicaid in states was linked to an increase in the unit reimbursement for nursing home services.[18]

The relationship of these two programs to the expansion of nursing home bed supply is elusive and confusing. Dunlop points out that the implementation of Medicare and Medicaid did not lead immediately to expanded nursing home bed complements. Rather, growth in the bed complement accelerated during the early 1960s, and actually *slowed* in the first full four years of Medicaid and Medicare. From 1963 to 1966, the bed supply grew at an annual rate of 10.7 percent. During 1967–70, the first full four years of Medicare, the rate slowed by half, to an annual growth rate of 5.4 percent. From 1971 to 1973 the rate accelerated to 8.3 percent, and subsided again slightly during the 1973–79 period.[19] The reduced growth rate in the first four years may have reflected industry concerns about the stability of the federal commitment to funding long-term care.

The relationship of Medicaid funding levels for nursing home care to the supply of beds is a subject of considerable controversy. Because of the near monopsonistic position of Medicaid in the nursing home market, William J. Scanlon believes that the rate paid by Medicaid is the principal rate limiter in the growth of nursing home supply. Scanlon conducted an extensive empirical analysis of the market for nursing home services using data from two years, 1969 and 1973. He performed several tests of hypotheses related to the presence of excess demand for nursing home services and demonstrated "the strong likelihood of considerable excess demand for nursing home care."[20]

According to Scanlon, the market for nursing home care is divided into self-pay and Medicaid segments. There are powerful incentives for nursing home operators to seek out the self-pay patient, who pays higher rates, and to queue the Medicaid patient. State governments are compelled to trade off rate increases for nursing homes against other services, and more recently against tax relief, and have thus restrained rates paid to nursing homes. If Scanlon's analysis is correct, the impact of increasing Medicaid rates for nursing home care could be multiplicative, not merely additive, since the supply of beds would expand in response.

Critics of the nursing home industry have pointed out that nursing home operators have nevertheless been able to generate substantial return on equity while relying on Medicaid reimbursement for half of their income and they suggest that the nursing home industry could not have attracted the capital to virtually double its bed complement if it were losing money on more than half its patients. At least one prominent analysis has suggested that expansion and profitability in the nursing home field has occurred at the explicit expense of quality care. Bruce Vladeck in his *Unloving Care* suggests that for-profit nursing homes operations have traded off profits against the amenities of care, given the low reimbursement rates provided by Medicaid and the inattentive monitoring by licensing agencies.[21]

Health planners and state budget officials believe that nursing home demand will simply expand with supply and, through Certificate of Need and rate decisions, have been unwilling to encourage further growth in capacity. Nursing home occupancy rates approaching 90 percent nationally, and exceeding this level in large states like Illinois, certainly suggest, however, that there is no excess capacity in the industry at the present time.

The controversy over the adequacy of supply of nursing home services is exacerbated by evidence that large amounts of inpatient expense to the Medicaid and Medicare programs are incurred by patients ready to be discharged from hospitals but unable to be placed. The principal reasons for this relate to nursing home industry unwillingness to deal with Medicare red tape and the lengthening queue for Medicaid recipients. Several studies in Massachusetts found that more than 1,000 patients in Massachusetts hospitals were awaiting nursing home placement on any given day. Estimates of hospital costs incurred annually ranged up to $20 million for the state.[22] No nationwide estimates of the amount of such hospitalization are available, though anecdotal evidence suggests the costs could amount to as much as $100 million annually.

No one really knows what the universe of need for nursing home care is. A General Accounting Office report to Congress in 1978 suggested that nearly 3 million elderly needed nursing home care but were not receiving it.[23] This number is more than double that of individuals currently in nursing homes. Various experts in the field of gerontology place the number of elderly having some form of handicap or impairment which impedes independent living at between 14 and 17 percent of the total population of elderly (a range of between 3.4 and 4.2 million people).

Proponents of alternatives to nursing home care point out that people in nursing homes spend only 2 percent of their waking hours receiving direct medical or nursing treatment.[24] They cite studies showing that only 37 percent of a large population of nursing home residents needed full time care and that an additional 26 percent needed only "supervised living."[25] The issue of the continuum of care for chronic illness will be explored below. Suffice it to say that there appears to be considerable demand for some type of care of the impaired aged, a demand which will grow with the increasing elderly population. Proponents of various modes of care believe this translates into demand for the services their organizations provide.

The proprietary presence in the nursing home industry

Unlike the hospital industry, for-profit providers of care dominate the nursing home industry. As of 1977, the latest year for which this type of data is available, 76.8 percent of the nursing home beds, 69.3 percent of the establishments, and 68.2 percent of the patients in nursing homes were in proprietary facilities.[26] By comparison, only about 60 percent of nursing home residents were in proprietary facilities in 1964.[27] Prior to the enactment of Medicaid, the vast majority of these proprietary facilities were of the type described above—small, family run operations housed in converted residences. However, since the middle 1960s, investor-owned firms have moved into nursing home administration. By 1979, these firms have grown in market position to an estimated 12 percent of all nursing home beds, a percentage roughly comparable to that of the management firms in the hospital industry. The total number of nursing home beds managed by these firms grew from approximately 149,000 in 1978 to almost 169,000 in 1979.[28] Perhaps because of the proprietary influence in the industry, it has been unusually susceptible to charges of profiteering and exploitation of patients. There were major nursing home scandals in New York State and elsewhere in the mid-1970s which damaged the industry's reputation.

In his analysis of nursing home efficiency, Michael Koetting found that, on the average, proprietary homes were more likely to be of lower quality than non-profit facilities and observed that

> the last decade has illustrated abundantly that proprietary institutions often have lower standards for appropriate levels of service provision and are much more likely to abuse existing procedures.[29]

However, research findings suggest that proprietary providers may well be more efficient than their nonprofit counterparts. Koetting found that "proprietary nursing homes are more efficient than nonprofit homes. Specifically, at any given quality level, proprietaries are less expensive. This is true even if allowance is made for a return on investment in proprietaries."[30] No data exists, however, on the relative efficiency of multi-unit versus freestanding for-profit homes.

High capital costs and cash flow difficulties from Medicaid and Medicare may be two major reasons why the investor-owned firms will continue to grow as a percentage of all nursing home operators. Like their hospital management counterparts, these firms have access to credit and, in some cases, equity markets which their nonprofit competitors do not. Koetting points out that "it does not seem likely that there is sufficient capital or management expertise in the nonprofit sector to expand to meet the rising demand for nursing home care."[31]

As in the hospital industry, the most rapid mode of expansion of the firms in the immediate future may be through management contracting or leasing rather than through direct ownership. Beds under contracts by management firms rose 28 percent from 1978 to 1979, and those under lease by 20 percent compared to a 5 percent growth in owned beds during the same period.[32]

Several of the large hospital management firms are developing a major presence in nursing homes as well. National Medical Enterprises acquired the third largest nursing home operator in the country, Hillhaven Corporation, in early 1980. Both Hospital Affiliates International, a subsidiary of the INA Corporation, and American Medical International have large nursing home operations as well. The nursing home industry giant is ARA Services, Incorporated, which controlled more than 31,000 beds in 1979 through four divisions.[33]

HOME HEALTH CARE AND THE ALTERNATIVES TO INSTITUTIONAL CARE

Unlike the acute end of the health care system, where patient care is mediated by the patient's physician, the chronic care end suffers from the lack of informed mediation between the patient and the system. As Scanlon points out in his analysis of the nursing home market, demand for long-term care and chronic care is not derived, but rather direct, demand. The patient and family are left to seek care amid a confusing array of possible alternatives. The confusion is heightened by shifting and inconsistent guidelines for eligibility and reimbursement for many services, and by a serious lack of information about the range of costs and types of care available.

At this point the principal competition of the nursing home is the burgeoning field of home health care services. Home health care falls along the continuum of care between the medical and custodial care of the nursing home and the social services provided by traditional social agencies. The medical services which may be provided in the home by a visiting nurse or aide including nursing; medical assistance; medical social work; physical, occupational, and speech therapy; and medical supplies and equipment. The nonmedical services may include homemaker assistance, meals on wheels, visiting, and telephone reassurance, and escort and chore services.

The split between medical and nonmedical services is artificial, since the inability of the patient to perform any number of functions—including housekeeping, transportation to and from therapy in a hospital, and self-medication with prescription drugs, to list only a few examples—may necessitate either prolonged hospitalization or institutional care in a nursing home. Yet the split becomes critically important since the rigid funding categories of federal health and social services programs will permit only certain programs to pay for certain forms of home care.

Until the fall of 1980, when Medicare program guidelines for home health care were liberalized, such home health benefits as nursing home benefits were linked to a minimum 3-day hospital stay, and were limited to 60 visits per illness. Medicare limited the provision on nonskilled (e.g., non-nursing services) by providing them only where skilled in-home nursing care was also provided. Conversely, the Title XX Social Services program under social security will reimburse *only* for nonskilled services. It takes prodigious energy and savvy to be able to coordinate funding from these various sources to provide enough of the right kinds of home care to individuals who need it.

In part because of the fragmentation at the federal and state levels, data on the amount and nature of home health services currently being provided to U.S. citizens is almost impossible to obtain. An Arthur Young study in mid-1980 estimated the size of the home health market to be $2.5 billion.[34] Data on government funding of home services during fiscal year 1977 revealed total spending of approximately $1 billion from the three programs involved. Medicare and

Medicaid financed home care for approximately 738,000 persons while Title XX paid for services for more than 1.6 million. The two groups may overlap considerably. Trend data on expenditures for Medicaid and Medicare show major growth in funding during the middle 1970s.

Medicare outlays for home health services have grown from $56.8 million in calendar year 1971 to $458 million in fiscal year 1977. At the time of this writing, fiscal 1979 outlays were estimated to be approximately $634 million. If this estimate is accurate, Medicare spent almost twice as much on home health care as it did on nursing home services during fiscal 1979. There is apparently considerable room for further expansion.

Research findings on the cost implications of home care have established that it can be important in forestalling hospitalization for certain patients as well as in reducing the length of hospitalization. Studies have been inconclusive on the relative cost effectiveness of home care relative to nursing home care. In his review of research literature on this point, John Hammond concluded:

> From the standpoint of third party underwriters, home health care is indeed less expensive than extended hospitalization. The limited number of articles available for review dictates caution in drawing a similar conclusion regarding the effect of home care on unnecessary hospital admissions. Available information indicates that the costs of home health services for patients requiring the same level of care are roughly equivalent to the cost of nursing home care.[35]

A problem with many cost studies may be the failure to factor in the cost of self care in the home. Costs to the *patient* (as opposed to the insurer) of in-home versus nursing home services can only be assessed if total living costs, not merely medical costs, are subjected to comparisons.

In his somewhat more thorough review of the literature on home health care costs and potential substitution for more costly modes of care, Avedis Donabedian is considerably more cautious than Hammond. In one study he reported that:

> [H]ome care was successful in managing the patients' heart disease, and was also instrumental in uncovering additional ill-

ness for which hospital care was necessary. Thus, the substitutive effect of the home care benefit was more than offset by the "discovery effect" of these same benefits, at least in this group of elderly and seriously ill patients. Once again, we find confirmation of the aphorism that "a little medical care breeds more medical care."[36]

Donabedian found confirmation of this effect in another study of cardiac patients as well as in two carefully controlled studies of attitudes of patients being discharged from chronic disease hospitals. He speculates that this discovery effect may be less pronounced for less seriously ill patients with self-limiting conditions or for less intensive home care. To the extent that the discovery effect prevails, cost advantages of home care could be reduced or even eliminated. These studies are part of the reason why insurers have moved cautiously in extending home care benefits.

Not a great deal is known about the competitors in this rapidly growing field. Data gathered from the Medicare program in Health and Human Services showed evidence of trends among competing providers of home health services. These can be seen in Figure 3–5.

Specifically, the number of participating Visiting Nurse Association agencies, the traditional provider of home care, declined by about 8 percent during the ten-year reporting period while the number of hospital-based programs participating in Medicare increased by 60 percent and the proprietary agencies by 268 percent. The number of proprietary providers had risen to 184 by the 1980 Arthur Young & Company report. This number underrepresents the actual number of proprietary home health providers. Until the 1980 program changes, federal statutes required proprietary providers to be licensed by a state agency in order to receive Medicare reimbursement. Since only 24 states both license home health agencies and permit proprietary operations, agencies in the remaining 26 states could not be reimbursed by Medicare. The elimination of the state licensure/certification requirement by federal law will substantially increase not only the number of participating agencies, but broaden access to home care in many states.

The number of hospital-based programs reported by Medicare may understate the actual number of hospital programs.

FIGURE 3-5
Participating Home Health Agencies, June 30, 1971–1980

Type	1971	1972	1973	1974	1975	1976	1980
Visiting nurses association	559	534	540	531	525	515	513
Combined government and voluntary	67	59	54	47	46	42	53
Official health agency	1,311	1,277	1,259	1,257	1,228	1,218	1,284
Rehabilitation based	12	11	11	10	9	10	6
Hospital based	209	219	244	267	273	280	335
Skilled nursing facility based	10	7	7	6	5	5	9
Proprietary	50	42	41	39	47	68	184
Other*	66	73	55	91	109	223	470
Total	2,284	2,222	2,211	2,248	2,242	2,361	2,854

* A majority of agencies in this category are private nonprofit.

Source: The information was made available by the Bureau of Health Insurance, Social Security Administration, HEW, to the Council of Home Health Agencies and Community Health Services, National League for Nursing. It appeared in *Community Home Health News*, December 1976, p. 3; 1980 data obtained from "Home Health: An Industry Composite" (Chicago: Arthur Young & Company 1980), p. 7. Reprinted by permission from the National League of Nursing.

By 1980 almost 350 hospitals offered home care services under Medicare, an increase of almost one third in four years. Total participating agencies had increased to more than 2,800. The Arthur Young study estimated that an additional 2,000 agencies offered home care services but, for a number of reasons, did not participate in Medicare.[37]

Though the growth of home health care services represents a potentially positive development from a cost standpoint, there may be other benefits to avoiding institutionalization which are difficult to quantify. These benefits include the psychological advantages accruing to a person who is supported in his or her effort to remain independent, and assistance to the families of elderly or seriously ill individuals who may themselves lack the medical or other capacity to maintain their family member at home. There is support in the literature for the efficacy of home care. Wan, Weissert and Livieratos reported that

> the use of day care and homemaker services can help the disabled elderly to sustain, if not to improve, their functioning. More specifically, the treatment modalities, day care and homemaker services, had an effect on the survivorship of patients, a positive effect on physical and mental well-being, and a limited but positive effect on social activity.[38]

The hidden agenda of policymakers who advocate expansion of home care benefits may be to strengthen the ability of elderly persons' families to care for them directly rather than placing them in nursing homes. The presence of nurses and home care aides in the home on a regular basis frees other family members for work or schooling while keeping the elderly person in the family environment. Nursing home operators have begun reinforcing home care by offering something called "respite care"—short-term institutionalization to permit family members to take vacations or do other things they would be unable to do with the elderly person at home. This is an excellent marketing tactic since it establishes the home's credibility for later, longer term institutional care. By reinforcing the family through home care, policymakers hope that long-term institutionalization can be avoided later.

Policymakers and social services advocates believe that home care represents an alternative to further major expansion of nursing home services as well as to costly hospitalization. The 1980 liberalization of benefits under Medicare is likely to expand care in this sector more rapidly than nursing home care over the next several years.

THE HOSPICE CONCEPT

Yet another alternative mode of providing care has emerged specifically for treatment of the terminally ill. The current organization of health care does not accommodate easily to the needs of the terminally ill, since it is organized, for the most part, around a high technology assault on acute illness. As initially developed by health care pioneer Dr. Cicely Saunders of St. Christopher's Hospice in London, the hospice concept involved providing spiritual and psychosocial help for the patient as well as palliative care to relieve the pain of terminal illness (primarily, but not exclusively, cancer), and bereavement counseling for the family. The approach is multidisciplinary, involving physicians, nursing and social services personnel, and priests and chaplains. Care is intended to be continuous, in contrast to the episodic course of treatment for most illness.

The movement grew rapidly during the 1970s. While only 3 hospices were in existence in the United States in 1975, there were 78 in operation only three years later, with more than 200 more in some stage of planning. The concept is not specific to a particular institutional setting. There are at least five possible ways of providing hospice care:

1. Hospice care in the home.
2. Hospice teams in hospitals.
3. Palliative care units in hospitals.
4. Hospital affiliated hospice programs.
5. Freestanding, autonomous hospices.[39]

The link to a hospital and to a primary physician, usually an oncologist (cancer specialist) is essential. Yet, hospice care is not necessarily an offset to inpatient hospital care as much as a different way of providing care. Thus it is impossible to speculate about the potential impact of this movement upon the demand for inpatient hospital services, other than to suggest that some people who die in hospitals might, for reasons of personal adjustment and concern for the impact on their families, choose to die at home or in other more supportive settings.

The key factor in determining the growth of this movement will be decisions by the major insurers including, ultimately, Medicare and Medicaid, concerning the insurability of hospice care. A number of pilot programs are being conducted by Blue Cross which will determine its future policy regarding reimbursement for hospice care.[40] At least one published study from the Blue Cross investigations does appear to support the cost effectiveness of a hospice program which heavily emphasized home care.[41] Until the results are in, acceptance of these programs as part of health insurance benefits packages is going to be cautious. Two large Blue Cross-insured industrial employers, General Electric and Westinghouse, did conclude contracts with Blue Cross to cover hospice benefits beginning in 1980.[42] It will take several years before the results of the debate regarding the merits of this new form of care are reflected in incentives to develop such services, but the concept appears to be promising.

THE PROBLEM OF COORDINATION

As mentioned above, the physician's responsibility for mediating aftercare for the patient is either attenuated or nonexistent. The declining role of the physician in managing chronic care and the disabilities associated with aging leaves the patient and his or her family essentially on its own in dealing with the variety of options available, except where the family is indigent or otherwise has access to a social caseworker.

The alternatives array themselves along a continuum of long-term care which runs from the institutional setting through a variety of ambulatory services to the home. The institution may be a hospital or a nursing home. Health policymakers and health care entrepreneurs are engaged in a lively debate, which has been underway since before the inception of Medicare and Medicaid, over the merits of choosing care at various points along this continuum. How services are used and in what mixture and for which problems and under whose supervision—these problems have yet to be solved adequately.

A solution of sorts appears to be in the making, however, in the form of fixed restraints. Medicaid and perhaps ultimately Medicare as well appear headed for periods of restrained growth. Thus, the resources devoted to long-term care may be capped by the necessity of restraining overall costs of these programs. This restraint will compel trade-offs not only between inpatient care and aftercare (which is much less expensive), but between the various forms of aftercare, which vary in cost (at least to the government). The search for "brokers" may extend beyond the acute care setting into aftercare as well.

A promising experiment which interposed a caring "honest broker" between providers of long-term care and elderly clients has been conducted in Connecticut to address the cost and access problems identified above. Triage Incorporated is a social agency supported by a demonstration grant from the Health Care Financing Administration (HCFA).[43] The agency serves the needs of elderly persons in a seven-town region of central Connecticut. Triage conducts an assessment of each elderly person and arranges for services needed *and* takes responsibility for purchasing them. The assessment is conducted by a team consisting of a nurse clinician and a social worker. HCFA granted Medicare waivers to reimburse through Triage for a variety of services not conventionally reimbursed by the program, including many home care social services, (homemaker, meals on wheels), intermediate care (institutional), legal services, and mental health counseling.

Triage was successful in navigating the range of available services for its clients. For 1,747 clients served in fiscal year 1978, Triage was able to save 81,275 long-term care days, at a net savings (net of Triage expenses) of $1.6 million, even including the cost of waivered services. That is, through the judicious use of alternative, non-institutional services, Triage was able to avoid 46.5 days of nursing home care per client per year, at an average annual savings to Medicare of almost $1,000 per elderly person. This amount represented an approximate 20 percent savings below costs which would have been incurred without the coordination. A key to the program is combining coordination of the service with payment for it. The increased clout given the coordinating agency was an important reason for the efficiency of the project. Decision-making about patient needs was placed in the hands of a concerned but fiscally responsible intermediary other than the provider of care.

THE ROLE OF THE HOSPITAL IN
THE AFTERCARE MARKET

As discussed above, hospitals have been getting out of the business of aftercare. In the last 25 years the long-term care patient day production of general hospitals has declined by almost 50 percent.[44] The withdrawal of the hospital from aftercare, in a period of rapid specialization of chronic and long-term care, has helped create some of the vacuum discussed above. Hospitals are intimately linked to the aftercare system through their social services departments. Caught between the pressures of professional standards review organizations to reduce the length of stay for Medicare patients and the tightness of nursing home bed supply, many hospitals are, perhaps against their wills, providing the missing coordination through their placement policies.

In an area growing and diversifying as rapidly as the aftercare market, there are exceptional opportunities for the hospital to broaden its service offerings. Until reimbursement questions are resolved, diversification into aftercare is likely to be a risky proposition. But aftercare does represent an opportunity for creative extension of the hospital's service mission to a population of elderly that will wield increasing economic and political power in the future, and whose needs are being inadequately met by the existing fragmented system.

One of the most interesting areas of potential diversification is the area of day hospitalization (or day care) for the geriatric patient. For the disabled or otherwise impaired elderly who are nonetheless ambulatory, day hospitalization can provide the mixture of health care, social service, and nutritional monitoring and assistance which many elderly receive in nursing homes. Such programs may fill the gap for that large segment of the nursing home population which does not require continuous nursing care. While the cost of adult day care is slightly higher on a per diem basis than nursing home care, preliminary study results suggest that it is from 37 to 60 percent less expensive to the payer, and between 12 and 35 percent less costly to the patient (when nonprogram expenses of independent living are added in), because it is intermittent rather than continuous care.[45]

The establishment of geriatric day care programs in hospitals permits the hospital to build from an institutional base which includes nursing and social services departments and to reprogram potentially under-utilized space to meet new needs. Hospitals with transportation systems can use them to transport patients to and from the hospital, expanding access to the program for those elderly who cannot drive and who live alone. Patients discharged from the hospital can be enrolled in the program.

The geriatric day care model can also be adapted to a community-based setting where the patients are drawn from the community at large rather than from the population of discharged patients. Many community health centers or primary care centers have the capability of adding geriatric day care programs to their mix of services, again without substantial alterations in staffing or mission.

As discussed above, many hospitals offer their own home health care services, which may range from traditional visiting nurse programs to such social services as homemakers and meals on wheels. The liberalization of Medicare home health benefits provides an economic opportunity for hospitals to expand these service offerings. Captive hospital-based home health care programs are cost reimbursed like most other hospital services, requiring a minimal alteration of billing and record-keeping procedures.

While research findings regarding the discovery effect of monitoring of patient conditions through home care may trouble insurers, they point to a marketing opportunity for hospitals to identify unmet health care needs. Not all of these needs can or should be met through hospitalizing the patient. But legitimate medical problems discovered through captive home health care programs can be treated somewhere within the orbit of the hospital's programs, either on an ambulatory or inpatient basis. Hospitals should be able to offer a full enough range of services to the elderly so that home health workers, in cooperation with the patient's physician, can select the most appropriate and, hopefully, least expensive means of solving medical problems identified through home care.

Even for hospitals which lack the capability or interest in developing captive aftercare programs, possibilities exist for making the hospital the broker between the patient and the bewildering array of alternative services for aftercare. This brokering role is being played already, but without the linkage for fiscal accountability which was established as critical in the Triage demonstration project. The University of Chicago Medical Center, through its social services department, is participating in an experiment which permits the hospital to serve as a clearing house for homemaker and chore/housekeeping services for a consortium of hospitals on the south side of Chicago. This model places on the referring hospital social worker responsibility for assessment of the hospitalized patient and the development of the in-home care services plan. It is responsible for selection and monitoring of home health providers, and for submitting claims to the reimbursing agency. This brokering function will help protect the patient as well as reduce medically unnecessary prolonged patient stays or re-admission, and will help divert as many patients as practical from the nursing home. Thus even where hospitals may not elect to develop their own aftercare programs, they can work with reimbursing agencies to coordinate the provision of aftercare services for their patients.

Through diversification into ambulatory and in-home care for the elderly hospitals can take advantage of their resource and administrative bases to help fill some of the vacuum of fragmentation and lack of accountability discussed above. The linkage to the patient's physician is preserved through such arrangements, and creative means of extending the physician responsibility for chronic care for the elderly through the hospital's nursing and social services staff will help preserve physician accountability for care, a critically missing link in much of the aftercare market.

NOTES

1. Anne Somers, "Rethinking Health Policy for the Elderly: A Six Point Program," *Inquiry*, Spring 1980, p. 12.
2. Charles Fisher, "Differences by Age Groups in Health Care Spending," *Health Care Financing Review*, Spring 1980, p. 66.
3. Ibid., p. 68.
4. Ibid., p. 81.
5. Somers, "Rethinking Health Policy for the Elderly," p. 3.
6. Ibid.
7. William J. Scanlon, "A Theory of the Nursing Home Market," *Inquiry*, Spring 1980, p. 25.
8. American Hospital Association, *Hospital Statistics* (Chicago: American Hospital Association, 1980), p. 6.
9. Burton Dunlop, *The Growth of Nursing Home Care* (Lexington, Mass.: Lexington Books, 1979), p. 29.
10. William Pollak, "Utilization of Alternative Care Settings by the Elderly," in *Community Planning for an Aging Society: Designing Services and Facilities*, M. Powell Lawton, Robert J. Newcomer, and Thomas O. Byerts, eds. (Stroudburg Pa.: Downden, Hutchinson and Ross, Incorporated, 1976), p. 114.
11. Ibid., p. 116.
12. Dunlop, *Growth of Nursing Home Care*, p. 40.
13. American Hospital Association, *Hospital Statistics*, pp. 5–6.
14. Dunlop, *Growth of Nursing Home Care*, p. 47.
15. House Select Committee on Aging Hearings, 1980, "Cutbacks in the Medicare Nursing Homes Programs," p. 3.
16. Dunlop, *Growth of Nursing Home Care*, p. 76.
17. Ibid., p. 67.
18. Ibid., p. 78.
19. Ibid., p. 7.
20. William J. Scanlon, "A Theory of the Nursing Home Market," *Inquiry*, Spring 1980, p. 34.
21. Bruce Vladeck, *Unloving Care* (New York: Basic Books, 1980).
22. Joan Dietz, "Useless Hospitalizations Cited in Reports of Nursing Home Beds," *Boston Globe*, May 3, 1979.
23. General Accounting Office Report to the Congress, "Entering a Nursing Home Costly Implications for Medicaid and the Elderly," November 26, 1979, pp. 26 ff.
24. Josephine Lee and Mary Stein, "Eliminating Duplication in Home Health Care for the Elderly: The Guale Project," *Health and Social Work*, 1980, p. 29.
25. William Weissert, "Costs of Adult Day Care: A Comparison to Nursing Homes," *Inquiry*, March 1978, p. 10.
26. United States Department of Health and Human Services Public Health Service Office of Health Research, Statistics and Technology National Center for Health Statistics, "The National Nursing Home Survey: 1977 Summary for the United States," series 13, no. 43.
27. United States Department of Health and Human Services, Public Health Services, Office of Health Research, Statistics and Technology, "Health

United States 1979," December 1980, DHHS Publication no. (PHS) 81–1232, p. 196.

28. Vince DiPaolo, "Tight Money, Higher Interest Rates Slow Nursing Home Growth," *Modern Healthcare,* June 1980, p. 76.

29. Michael Koetting, *Nursing Home Organization and Efficiency,* (Lexington, Mass.: Lexington Books, 1980), p. 100.

30. Ibid., p. 99.

31. Ibid.

32. DiPaolo, "Tight Money, Higher Interest Rates Slow Nursing Home Growth," p. 84.

33. Ibid., p. 76.

34. Arthur Young and Company, "Home Health: An Industry Composite," New York: Arthur Young and Company, August 1980), p. 2.

35. John Hammond, "Home Health Care Cost Effectiveness: An Overview of the Literature," *Public Health Reports,* 94, no. 41 (July–August 1979): 311.

36. Avedis Donabedian, *Benefits in Medical Care Administration* (Cambridge, Mass.: Harvard University Press, 1976), p. 79.

37. Arthur Young and Company, "Home Health: An Industry Composite."

38. Thomas Wan, William Weissert, and Barbara Livieratos, "Geriatric Day Care and Homemaker Services: An Experimental Study," *Journal of Gerontology* 35, no. 2 (1980): 273.

39. Florence Wald, Zelda Forster, and Henry Wald, "The Hospice Movement as a Health Care Reform," *Nursing Outlook,* March 1980, pp. 173–74.

40. "Survival of Hospices Depends on Insurers," *Modern Healthcare,* November 1980, p. 58.

41. Ibid.

42. Ibid.

43. "Long-Term Care for the 1980's: Channeling Demonstrations and Other Initiatives," hearing before the Subcommittee on Health and Long-term Care, Washington, D.C., February 27, 1980, p. 19.

44. See Figure 3–3.

45. William Weissert, "Costs of Adult Day Care: A Comparison to Nursing Homes," *Inquiry,* March 1978, p. 17.

4 Health maintenance

The third sector which promises to impinge on the core inpatient market of the nation's hospitals is comprised of those hybrid health insurance plan/delivery systems popularly known as health maintenance organizations (HMOs).* As will be established below, the principal economic consequences of the HMO involve lowering hospital utilization and rates through brokering of health care for HMO enrollees. As such, HMO development is targeted at restraining hospital use and costs. The strength of the health maintenance concept may be its flexibility—the ability to adapt to different physician, employer, and community perceptions and needs. Fee-for-service medicine, private office practice, and third party insurance, as well as free physician choice, can all be encompassed within the alternative delivery system, while still retaining certain core features of health maintenance.

---

* Advocates of HMOs have urged relabelling them "alternative delivery systems," an unendearing expression intended to encompass more types of organizations than the closed panel staff or group HMO.

The health maintenance organization is a controversial enterprise. Like group practice, it has been subjected to attack by organized medicine and for many of the same reasons (compromising physician autonomy, threatening quality of medical care, etc.). It has equally zealous supporters who claim that this model, if supported by changes in tax and insurance laws, can help solve the nation's health cost crisis. It is difficult to make an objective assessment of the HMO without being accused of bias by at least one side of the debate. However, the debate itself is one of the healthiest developments in health care, and the results may influence national health policy significantly during the 1980s.

WHAT IS A HEALTH MAINTENANCE ORGANIZATION?

The health maintenance concept grew out of successful models of prepaid group practice, the largest and best known of which is the Kaiser/Permanente Group Plan of California, founded during the 1930s. Health maintenance organizations are prepaid a fixed fee by enrollees which covers a full range of medical services from routine office visits to hospitalization. Because the HMO encompasses ambulatory as well as inpatient care, it is a vertically integrated health enterprise. The same entity which collects the fees from enrollees provides them care. In a few cases (notably Kaiser), this integration may extend to ownership of the hospitals in which HMO patients receive inpatient care. More typically, HMOs contract with hospitals in their communities for care. In the vast majority of HMOs the concept of insurance, or third party payment, plays a much reduced role. Physician services are provided by groups of physicians who are either incorporated separately as a group practice and sell their services to the HMO on a per capita basis (the group model), or by staff physicians who are salaried employees of the HMO (the staff model).

The essence of health maintenance is that the health care provided to the enrolled population is *managed,* within fixed predictable resource limits, by the HMO. Enthoven has likened the management role of the HMO to that of a prime contractor in arranging comprehensive care for its patients. The HMO thus assumes at least part of the role traditionally occupied by the physician under traditional fee-for-service practice. The prime contractor feature of health maintenance organizations is at the economic heart of competitive health care proposals put forward by health maintenance advocates. HMOs will seek out the most efficient providers of care, often through competitive bidding. HMOs thus become economic brokers for their enrollees, offering hospitals and other providers large blocs of utilization in exchange for a good price.

Competitive models rest upon the growth of this brokering function to compel established providers to be more efficient. In this competitive system, hospitals will not necessarily be paid their "reasonable costs" for rendering care to groups of plan enrollees; rather they will be paid what they can get. How much "brokering" is required in a given hospital market to effect overall costs is a subject of ongoing research, and is the "$64,000 Question" about health maintenance.

At the same time, since sickness is a cost to the HMO the financing mechanism contains incentives both to improve health status (through screening, physical examinations, and other preventive health measures), and to minimize use of expensive health services such as hospital care. HMO proponents believe that the fee-for-service system encourages cost increasing behavior by rewarding the physician for each intervention. Because HMOs reverse this incentive, proponents argue they save money. Physicians participating in HMOs are unquestionably subject to stricter oversight of their practice than private practice colleagues, including, in many cases, prior authorization of hospital admissions.

Several variations on the prepaid group practice model have emerged in response to market and, some speculate, political pressures. The most popular variation is the Independent Practice Association (IPA), which contracts with physicians who practice in their own offices to render care to enrolled patients. As with the conventional prepaid group practice HMO, the IPA is responsible for providing a comprehensive range of health services for its enrollees. Its physicians comingle enrollees with their private patients (typically not more than 15 percent of an IPAs physician's patients are enrolled in the plan), and are compensated for their services on a fee-for-service basis. However, the fees may be paid on the basis of a negotiated fee schedule limiting maximum reimbursement. Fee reimbursement may also be reduced below these negotiated levels if the plan experiences financial difficulty. Physicians are also subject to peer review of their hospital utilization practices. The principal attraction of the IPA for potential enrollees is that they typically involve a large enough percentage of the physicians practicing in an area to guarantee potential enrollees their choice of physician or, implicitly, the continued services of their family doctor. As will be seen later, this feature may be pivotal to the ultimate market prospects and penetration of the HMO.

A third variation is the primary care network (PCN). This type of organization pioneered by the SAFECO Insurance firm is a coalition between a private health insurer and contracting primary physicians (internists, family practitioners). The participating physicians, who are reimbursed for their services by the insurance company on a capitation (per capita) basis, are responsible for arranging all care for their patients. What services they cannot supply themselves they arrange through referral. The cost of referral services and hospitalization are picked up by the insurance company from the pool of fees paid by enrollees. If the pool runs a surplus it is split with the physician. If it runs a deficit a portion of the deficit is reduced through reduced fee payments, putting the physician at risk financially for routine care. Catastrophic hospitalization costs are paid by the insurance company. Here the physician becomes a financially responsible intermediary for the insurance company in arranging care.

All these methods have in common an alteration of the economic relationship between the doctor and patient in such a way that the physician is encouraged to avoid, to the extent medically and ethically permissable, using expensive medical services in caring for the patient. The spectrum of control ranges from the physician being a salaried employee of the plan (staff-type HMO) to the physician being a mildly constrained independent contractor (IPA). In all these arrangements peer or corporate control is exercised to some degree over the practice habits of participating physicians. In all cases such participation by the physician is voluntary.

HMO AND COST CONTROL

An extensive body of research has established that the total health cost to the consumer of HMO care, at least under the prepaid group practice mode, is lower than can be rendered under competing fee-for-service insurance plans. It is important to realize that these results relate not to premium costs (the cost of insurance benefits) but to the total cost of care, including out-of-pocket outlays. This is an important distinction because enrollment fees for HMOs are often higher than for conventional group health insurance premiums. But because they cover more services and do not contain deductibles or co-insurance, overall outlays for care are lower in HMOs.

According to Harold S. Luft, who summarized about 50 comparative studies of HMO costs relative to conventional group health insurance, total health costs to HMO subscribers range from 10 to 40 percent below those of subscribers to comparable group insurance plans.[1] This specific finding ties to research conducted in California, where the HMO cost data derives from the very large, established Kaiser HMO network. Whether these cost reductions will be duplicated by the large cohort of newer HMOs started up during the 1970s remains to be determined.

With regard to IPAs, Luft could find no evidence that costs to enrollees in them were lower than for conventional insurance.[2] This latter finding is potentially significant since it could be argued that the IPA concept has traded away cost reducing features of prepaid group practice to accommodate the fee-for-service system. That is, physician behavior may not be sufficiently altered by the IPA to influence his or her pattern of use of expensive services.

Luft's review establishes conclusively that HMO cost savings are attributable directly to lower rates of hospitalization of enrolled patients. Specifically, research has found that hospital inpatient days are from 25 to 40 percent lower for HMO enrollees and from 0 to 25 percent lower for IPAs than for comparison groups of the conventionally insured.[3] The National HMO Census taken in 1980 estimated that HMOs nationwide generated only 418 patient days of care per 1,000 population. This compares to a nationwide average of 1,235 days per 1,000 population. The relative degree of hospital use varies according to HMO type, with "group" HMOs below the mean and IPA's 20 to 30 percent above the mean.[4]

Inpatient bed days are the product of two factors: admissions and length of stay. While Luft found that length of stay does not appear to be shorter for HMO patients, the rate of hospital admissions appear to be lower for HMO patients. However, the AMA study of 15 HMOs did find systematically lower lengths of stay in HMOs compared with the same community's Blue Cross plan.[5] In attempting to tease this problem apart a little further, Luft searched for evidence that HMOs reduce discretionary admissions, such as elective surgery, and found no support for this hypothesis.

Luft established that HMOs do not achieve savings by reducing ambulatory care. In fact, 10 of the 17 non-IPA HMOs surveyed experienced higher rates of ambulatory use than paired groups of the conventionally insured. Of five IPAs in the studies Luft reviewed, all had substantially higher rates of ambulatory usage relative to conventionally insured group plans.

Though research has established the reasons why HMO care appears to result in lower health care costs, e.g., lower hospitalization rates, the underlying causes of the lower hospitalization rates are still a subject of controversy. HMO advocates claim that these lower rates are the results of a better organized system of care, more prevention, and other factors. HMO detractors claim that it is because the people who enroll in HMOs were unlikely to require hospitalization or expensive care in the first place, and that the system of care cannot claim responsibility.

These critics point to the fact that HMOs enroll only about 1.5 percent of the nation's more than 50 million Medicaid and Medicare recipients. Both of these groups are high risk medically and consume more (in the case of the elderly, *much* more) hospital care than the national average. The Interstudy HMO Census found that people over 65 comprised only 4.6 percent of total HMO enrollment. The average proportion of elderly enrollees among the AMA study sample of 15 HMO plans was 6.1 percent.[6] The elderly have a hospitalization rate more than triple that of the national average.

Proponents of the HMO concept agree that as the HMO enrollment base broadens the average rates of hospitalization will probably rise, and costs will rise along with them. Where this ultimate rise will place HMO costs relative to conventional health insurance plans such as Blue Cross remains to be seen.

THE MARKET FOR THE HMO

The most recent estimate of total HMO enrollment in the United States is the federal government's 1980 National HMO Census. As of June 1980 there were 9.1 million Americans enrolled in HMOs, 72 percent more than in 1974. Of this group, 1.3 million were enrolled in IPAs.[7] There were 236 HMOs, according to the survey, of which 34 percent were IPAs.[8] The Louis Harris poll regarding national attitudes toward HMOs conducted during the summer of 1980 established that approximately 6 percent of adult Americans were then enrolled in HMOs, but that there is sharp regional variation in HMO penetration. While 20 perent of all adults in the West are enrolled in HMOs, only 4 percent in the Midwest, 3 percent in the East, and 1 percent in the South are enrolled. The Harris poll also found that enrollments are higher in cities and suburbs than in rural areas and small towns.[9] The 1980 HMO Census conducted by the federal government also established that HMO enrollment is unevenly distributed in the national market. Nearly 59 percent of all HMO enrollment is in the West and 44 percent in the state of California.[10]

When one looks behind the enrollment data to the organizations themselves, one can see that, despite impressive growth in the number of HMOs since 1970, in enrollment terms, the market can still be characterized as "Kaiser/Permanente and everybody else." Kaiser plan enrollments, which are heavily concentrated in California and other western states, totalled 3.9 million in 1980, 42 percent of all HMO enrollment. Kaiser accounts for approximately 75 percent of the enrollment of all HMOs which have met federal requirements for financial and marketing assistance. Of the 12 HMOs with enrollments over 100,000, five are Kaiser plans.[10] Blue Cross is also a significant institutional presence in the HMO field. Local Blue Cross sponsors 44 HMOs nationally and is assisting some 27 others.[11] The significance of this degree of involvement by large health insurers will be discussed below. See Figure 4–2.

The Harris poll found no significant differences in rates of enrollment by race, sex, marital status, or number of children in family under age 18. Those with college level education, income over $25,000, and those who work for very large organizations were over-represented in the enrolled population relative to other groups. Professionals are over-represented in the HMO enrollment data, while executive/proprietor and skilled labor groups were underrepresented.

Annual enrollment in HMOs grew by only 5 percent from 1976 to 1977, but increased by 18 percent from 1977 to 1978 and by 12 percent annually during the subsequent two years. Interestingly, 56 percent of the sharp 1977–78 growth in HMO enrollment occurred in IPAs. The IPA share of the HMO market appears to be growing relative to the other types of HMO. The proportion of HMOs that were IPAs grew from 25 to 34 percent from 1975 to 1978, while the proportion of HMO enrollment accounted for by IPAs grew from 6.5 to 14.1 percent from 1976 to 1978.[12]

The public opinion data gathered by Harris provide a clue to the underlying market issues responsible for the above pattern. Harris established that approximately 10 percent of the nonenrolled U.S. population was very interested in possible future HMO enrollment. However, this percentage *more than doubles* (to 26 percent) if non-members are informed that it may be possible to retain their family doctor.[13] The Harris survey concluded that the market for future HMO growth is limited (more than 58 percent of those polled were hardly or not at all interested[14]) and that the problem of breaking private physician ties (e.g., inability to choose the HMO physician) may be a major impediment to growth.

However, a more fundamental problem faces those who wish to expand HMO enrollment. That problem is that the vast majority of the general public simply does not understand what an HMO is, let alone what benefits it is likely to confer upon its members. Fully 79 percent of the general public indicated that they are either not very or not at all familiar with the HMO concept, while only 5 percent said they were very familiar with the concept.[15] This is not surprising since the concept itself and the differences between HMOs and conventional health insurance are quite complex. As Harris points out, it is difficult to market something to a population that does not understand the product or its potential benefits.

The key intermediary in HMO enrollment is the employer, not the consumer of health care. The vast majority of enrollees participate in HMOs as part of an employee health benefit package. Thus the real market for HMOs is the employer and the competition is other health insurance plans. HMOs are already at a disadvantage in this competition because, as Enthoven points out, premium costs (to the employer) of HMOs are likely to be higher for the first several years of an HMO than competing group health insurance plans. Only established plans like Kaiser are able to enter this competition on a relatively good footing.

The Federal HMO Act of 1973 requires employers to offer qualified HMOs as a benefit alternative if available in their area. This requirement has engendered isolated but angry resistance from some firms who resent federal mandates driving up their health benefits outlays. Harris correctly points out that the employer will have to bear much of the burden of educating the employee about the benefits of HMO membership relative to enrollment in more conventional health insurance plans. To the extent that employer vested interests in lower health care costs are a more prominent feature of the marketing effort than how HMOs can benefit the employee, these educational efforts may be rejected as "company medicine," much as industrial health care clinics have been in the past. This has been a particular problem with company based HMOs such as those advocated by Paul Ellwood in his well-known 1973 article "Health Care:

Should Industry Buy It or Sell It?"[16] The employer in such instances is hardly a disinterested participant in the process.

The Harris public opinion data provide some valuable clues to effective marketing strategies for the HMO manager. Figure 4–1 compares product attributes of HMO care relative to fee-for-service care according to users of each mode of care. Cost bulks the largest among the factors favoring HMOs—a complex issue since, as pointed out earlier, the cost differences may reflect much lower out of pocket outlays due to the comprehensiveness of HMO coverage, but higher upfront premium costs. The additional features of health education and prevention programs are unique attributes of

FIGURE 4–1
Levels of satisfaction with various aspects of available health care service: net difference between members and nonmembers

Q.: I would like you to tell me how satisfied you are with various elements of the health care services that are available to you and your family. Please say for each one whether you are very satisfied, somewhat satisfied, somewhat dissatisfied, or very dissatisfied.

	Net difference between percentage of members and nonmembers saying "very satisfied"
The cost to you and your family—not met by insurance—of health care services	+27
The Total cost—whether you pay for it yourself or not—of health care services	+23
The availability of doctors and medical services 24 hours a day, 7 days a week	+17
The availability of adequate preventitive health services	+15
The availability of health education for your family	+10
The amount of time you have to wait to see a doctor after you have called for an appointment	− 5
The helpfulness and general attitude of your doctors	− 8
Your ability to see a doctor whenever you need to	− 9
The quality of doctors	−12

Source: Reprinted with permission from Louis Harris and Associates, Inc. "American Attitudes Toward Health Care Maintenance Organizations" (Menlo Park, California: The Henry J. Kaiser Family Foundation, July 1980).

HMO care which fee-for-service medicine is not well organized to provide (except through some hospitals).

The negative attributes, unfortunately, relate to the core product—medical care. The perceived differences between HMO and fee-for-service care relative to both quality of and access to physicians are significant. Fully 30 percent of HMO users were dissatisfied both with the waiting time for a physician appointment and the waiting time once in the facility to see the physician. Perceived quality and attitudes of physicians in HMO settings were also significantly less favorable than in the fee-for-service settings. Unfortunately, this data did not differentiate between HMO users who saw their physicians in an IPA setting as against a group/staff HMO setting.

This consumer perception contradicts research findings, summarized by Frances Cunningham and John Williamson, which suggested that the quality of health care in HMOs, measured by a variety of empirical techniques, is superior to care rendered in other settings.[17] The difference between "objective" measures of quality and consumer perceptions suggests that HMOs have not done an effective job of differentiating their product from conventional modes of health care and, perhaps, have not paid as much attention to the amenities of care as they should.

The problems of accessibility and quality must be addressed forthrightly by HMO marketers because they represent two areas where HMOs are likely to have image problems in the future. The IPA has an obvious competitive advantage over the closed panel group or staff HMOs since patients are permitted to remain with physicians in whom they have confidence. In terms of accessibility, HMOs may be compelled to commit to maximum waiting times for appointments and to allocate appropriate resources to keep these commitments. They may also be bucking a consumer unwillingness to permit non-M.D. allied health personnel to assume a larger role in their health management. HMOs have been more aggressive in substituting nurse practitioners and physician assistants for physicians where possible (taking histories and conducting physicals, for example). The AMA study estimated that approximately 30 percent of all medical encounters in half of the non-IPA HMOs they studied are handled by allied health personnel.[18] As consumers accept the role of these personnel, demand for physician contact may subside somewhat.

Keeping management attention focused on the core issues of the perceived quality of service is difficult in many cases because most HMOs are new business ventures. Like all new ventures, HMOs are fragile, and maneuvering them out of the take-off phase is a complex, anxiety-ridden enterprise. Fourteen federal qualified HMOs have gone bankrupt in the last eight years, and many times this number may follow if the Reagan administration limits loans for HMO development.[19] These problems are aggravated by certain federal requirements for HMOs desiring federal support, such as required periods of open enrollment and the use of community rating for premiums rather than ratings related to individual health status. It may take $3 to $5 million of deficit and five to six years' time before a staff or group HMO reaches the breakeven point.*[20] Depending on the mix of services offered, it may take an enrollment of 30,000 to 40,000 to reach breakeven. IPAs usually take much less capital and a lower enrollment level to break even.[21] Financial management and marketing to employers may crowd out managing for consumer acceptance.

Estimating the likely rate of enrollment is the most complex methodological problem encountered in planning for the growth of the HMO. The most effective method of doing this is by estimating from a base of sponsoring institutions which may have themselves have studied the enrollment potential of their employee groups as part of their benefits planning process. Community surveys are not a cost-effective method of estimating potential markets, because they ignore the key mediating role of the employer in the HMO choice. Accurate estimates of enrollment are critical to the financial management of the HMO since these rates determine the projected revenue flow within which the HMO must live, given the level of upfront funding expected (federal loans,

---

* These estimates were derived from a 1974 study. Assuming that the underlying economics have not changed, these figures should be roughly *doubled* to reflect 1981 costs.

etc.). Available revenues govern staffing and other resource allocation decisions, in turn affecting the mix of services the HMO can offer. The problem which HMOs face in their first several years is in managing the deficit. Since these facilities are simultaneously struggling to gain consumer and employer acceptance, it is important that some type of feedback mechanism (patient satisfaction surveys or other less formal devices) be built into evaluation to assure that consumer needs are not sacrificed during the start-up period.

The growth rate of health maintenance organization enrollments in the future is uncertain. The Harris data suggest two reasons why growth will not be necessarily be rapid. The first is public ignorance of the HMO concept. The second is the relatively limited appeal of the HMO in a health care system where the vast majority of consumers have satisfactory physician relationships under fee-for-service. The loss of freedom of physician choice, and the implicit loss of choice of hospital which follows, is a significant market impediment to future growth. Finally, the consumer jury is still out on the implicit trade-offs in access and, possibly, quality of care. Since the HMO is still a relatively unknown quantity in the health care market, consumer skepticism will have to be countered by solid achievements in providing quality patient care.

As mentioned earlier, the rates of hospitalization within HMO populations are likely to rise as the base broadens. If the HMO is not able to reduce significantly the rates of utilization among newly recruited populations, including the medically indigent and the elderly, the cost advantage between the struggling community-based HMO and the established insurance plan will narrow and could disappear. Open enrollment and community rating (which inhibit selective enrollment of low-risk groups) will probably pull HMO medical care use and costs up, all other things being equal. The rate of increase in utilization and cost as HMO enrollment broadens will test the theory behind the HMO. The results of the test may bear directly on the marketability of the HMO.

Perhaps recognizing these significant uncertainties, HMO advocates have begun to analyze the competitive framework within which health insurers operate. A major feature of this competitive environment relates to the federal income tax exclusion of employer contributions to health benefits. This tax exclusion encourages employees to demand, through their unions, that employers pay the full cost of health insurance premiums, regardless of the total cost of care delivered under the plan. HMO advocates recognize that it may be difficult to reach the market share they seek if the groundrules for enrollment in health insurance programs are not tilted in the direction of greater employee choice (e.g., multiple plans) and greater economic "neutrality" respecting the type of plans offered.

Thus, rather than offer a single health benefit plan, Enthoven argues that employers should offer several, including prepaid health plans. Because of the tax exclusion mentioned above, however, Enthoven believes that multiple choice alone will not suffice to encourage competition among plans. He argues that the federal government should also establish conditions for continued exclusion of employer health benefit contributions from federal taxation. Specifically, only those plans which provide certain cost containment features should be permitted to receive the exemption. Finally, the employer contribution should be *fixed* at some level below the total premium cost of care so that the consumer, in choosing between competing health plans, is to some extent at economic risk in allocating his or her portion of the premium.

Under the present system the employer, not the employee, reaps the benefits of the employee's choice of a less expensive health care plan. Under a system of fixed contributions, the employee would bear the responsibility for economic choice and participate in the rewards. It is presumed that the changes in federal tax and employee benefits policies proposed, which are substantial, would create the correct mix of economic incentives to further growth of HMOs. Right now, the employer-group health insurance nexus is perceived by HMO advocates to be the principal barrier to the growth of alternative delivery systems.

Whether the far-reaching changes proposed by HMO advocates will be enacted by Congress remains to be seen. If HMOs are permitted to compete in the consumer rather than in the employer marketplace, some of the economic and product benefits of HMOs can enter more directly into the consumer decision, and HMOs may be able to achieve greater market penetration than under the current ground-rules. Without the changes, the market for alternative delivery systems is likely to remain limited, and probably will not exceed 10 percent of the U.S. population before 1990.

COMPETITIVE IMPLICATIONS OF ALTERNATIVE DELIVERY SYSTEMS

The health maintenance organization was endorsed by the Nixon administration as an innovative device for restraining health care cost increases by providing an alternative to the fee-for-service physician and the cost-reimbursed hospital systems. To the extent that HMOs are successful in penetrating the health care market, they will reduce the number of patients who are treated under fee-for-service reimbursement. Through brokering hospital care for large panels of enrollees through economic competition, as well as restraining aggregate hospital utilization, HMOs may also pull down hospital utilization and revenues and narrow profit margins. For these reasons, the HMO is a competitive problem for both the physician and the hospital.

When HMOs were first developed they were subjected to intense opposition from local medical societies. Participating physicians were sometimes censured or expelled from their local medical societies or denied hospital admitting privileges. Since the specter of antitrust has raised its head in the health care field, many overtly public anticompetitive practices of the past have gone underground or been abandoned. Rather, physician groups and medical societies have increasingly flocked to the IPA as an alternative to the closed panel, group, or staff HMO. Many IPAs are formed as a defensive measure by local physicians to assure their ability to keep their patients while permitting them access to prepaid care. Some HMO advocates have argued that there are antitrust implications of IPAs with 80 to 95 percent of the physicians in a county or city participating.

The research findings available so far suggest that the increased freedom of choice afforded the consumer by the

IPA has economic trade-offs. Specifically, the fee-for-service system remains in place. Findings which indicate higher levels of physician visits in IPAs relative to HMOs as well as higher rates of hospitalization, suggest that IPA cost reduction mechanisms and, implicitly, peer pressures, are not as effective as in closed panel HMOs. The IPA and the closed panel systems may be generically different. With growing physician supply, and multiple IPAs, these physician groups may begin competing among each other, tightening cost and utilization controls as a consequence. Recent marginal growth in HMO enrollment has been among IPAs.

The fee-for-service system, and the high level of consumer satisfaction with the care received under that system, is well entrenched and accepted by patients. Advocates of HMOs may be compelled by market realities to temper their desire for structural reform by encouraging pluralism among different methods of organizing prepaid care which incorporate fee-for-service practice. Under the type of system Enthoven advocates, however, the ultimate competitive outcome will be determined by the consumer, responding to systems of care which do the best job of meeting economic and medical needs.

The implications for the hospital are less clear. As discussed above, it is still not certain how much the HMO actually reduces the hospital utilization of its enrollees, as opposed to enrolling people who use less care already. To the extent that HMOs actually reduce the need for hospitalization, increased enrollment of HMOs in a community or market area will reduce the demand for hospital utilization in that area.

The impact on the hospital, and the posture the hospital takes toward the HMO, will depend on the strength of the hospital's market position. Hospitals with strong medical staffs and high utilization can probably ignore the HMO. Hospitals with marginal utilization are faced with two choices—ignore the HMO and hope that lost utilization will be absorbed by other institutions, or work with the HMO to sell it services. Depending on the financial circumstances of the hospital, it may be appropriate to bargain with the HMO to offer hospital services to its enrollees at a discount below the hospital's prevailing charges for services. Communities with a sufficient penetration of HMOs will probably experience bidding wars between hospitals attempting to secure HMO hospital utilization. How much the hospital system can "absorb" via competitive bidding without eating away net incomes will depend on the degree of management control over costs and on the collective market power of prepaid plans in the community.

Some larger hospitals have been involved in sponsoring health maintenance organizations as outreach strategies. Several of the larger teaching hospitals in the Chicago area have sponsored HMOs and established branches throughout the metropolitan area, including areas they may not have penetrated through their voluntary staffs. There are several good reasons for a hospital to sponsor an HMO, including possible reduction of its own health benefits costs and helping to participate in reform of the health care system.

However, hospital executives must understand the implications of the inherent conflict of interest between the HMO and the hospital before embarking on such a course. If a captive HMO is to meet its economic objectives and minimize its fee levels, there are powerful incentives to minimize reliance on the parent hospital and seek out less expensive hospital settings closer to the patient's home or to the HMOs outlets, as well as to bargain aggressively for lower rates for the services the captive does choose to purchase from the parent institution.

In addition, because the HMO delivers most of its care in an ambulatory setting and deals with a great amount of self-limiting disease, and because of the utilization controls the HMO imposes on hospitalization, the rate of admission of patients per quantum of HMO visits is likely to be far lower than from the hospital's own emergency room or outpatient clinics. Ellwood's estimate that it takes an HMO enrollment of 100,000 persons (which only 12 health care plans have yet achieved in the United States), to support a 200-bed hospital suggest that HMOs may not be an effective method of sustaining or increasing hospital use.

As far as the major actors in the HMO markets, there have thus far been four—hospitals, physician groups, community/employer based groups, and insurance companies.

Many HMOs started during the early 1970s were sponsored by community and employer organizations, though as mentioned above, IPA growth has increased in the last five years, as have insurance company sponsored plans. With the exception of insurance company based plans and Kaiser, these groups have tended to be under-capitalized, requiring reliance on federal grants and loan guarantees, and undermanaged, reflecting their inability in many cases to recruit competent personnel. Managing the start-up phases of any new venture is a difficult undertaking. For reasons mentioned above, hospitals are unlikely to form many additional HMOs. Federal funding is more likely to be withdrawn than to grow. To the extent that the field is to grow, it may be the insurance companies, including Blue Cross, and the hospital management firms that will be the dominant presence in the HMO market. These organizations have extraordinary access to capital, as well as extensive marketing expertise and access to corporate benefits programs.

HMOs owned or operated by large national firms currently account for about 60 percent of all HMO enrollment. A listing of HMOs owned or managed by national firms may be seen in Figure 4–2. If the federal government caps its loan guarantee program, as has been proposed in the fiscal year 1982 federal budget, further infusion of capital into this market

FIGURE 4–2
HMOs owned or managed by national firms

	Number of plans	Enrollment
Kaiser	8	3,876,000
Blue Cross	39*	782,000
INA	6	391,000
American Medical International	4	110,000
Charter Medical	5	103,000
Connecticut General	2	67,000
Prudential	4	48,000+
CNA	2	43,000
SAFECO	4	38,000
Total	74	5,447,000

* Does not count 30 which receive extensive technical and management assistance from Blue Cross.
+ Includes 11,000 in joint venture with Kaiser in Dallas, Texas.
Source: *Interstudy*, telephone conversation with Research Department.

will come from the private sector. In this case, penetration by the national firms will increase, making them the dominant force in the HMO sector.

This movement by the national firms, while a defensive strategy primarily, reflects sound corporate planning and a belief that the future profitability of their conventional lines of group health insurance may be compromised by growing employer resistance to passing through escalating health care costs. Insurance companies may be willing to diversify into alternative delivery systems to protect their market share and enrollment base, even at the price of substantial initial subsidies. They are by far the best capitalized potential actors in the system. Since HMOs deliver care as well as finance it, insurance industry entry into the health maintenance market moves them into the business of organizing and delivering health care. How far the insurance firms are willing to tread along this possible path of integration will be one of the most interesting developments to watch in the next 15 or 20 years.

NOTES

1. Harold S. Luft, "How Do Health Maintenance Organizations Achieve Their 'Savings'?" *The New England Journal of Medicine,* June 15, 1978, p. 1337.
2. Ibid., p. 1336.
3. Ibid.
4. American Medical Association Council on Medical Service Information, distributed as background data for the Council on Medical Services Report A (A-80): "Study of Health Maintenance Organizations," (Chicago: American Medical Association), p. 16.
5. Ibid.
6. Ibid., p. 15.
7. *Interstudy,* "July 1980 Survey Results: HMO Enrollment and Utilization in the U.S." (Excelsior, Minnesota: *Interstudy,* July 1980).
8. Ibid.
9. Louis Harris and Associates, "American Attitudes toward Health Maintenance Organizations" (Menlo Park, California: The Henry J. Kaiser Family Foundation, July, 1980, p. 13.
10. United States Department of Health and Human Services, "National HMO Census, 1980" (Washington, D.C.: Public Health Service, 1980), p. 2.
11. Blue Cross/Blue Shield Association, telephone conversation with Department of Alternative Delivery Systems, July 24, 1981.
12. John K. Iglehart, "HMO's—An Idea Whose Time Has Come?" *National Journal,* February 25, 1978, p. 314.

13. Harris and Associates, "American Attitudes toward Health Maintenance Organizations," p. 4.
14. Ibid.
15. Ibid., p. 20.
16. Paul M. Ellwood, Jr. and Michael E. Herbert, "Health Care: Should Industry Buy It or Sell It?" *Harvard Business Review,* July–August, 1973, p. 99.
17. Frances Cunningham and John Williamson, M.D. "How Does the Quality of Health Care in HMOs Compare to That in Other Settings? An Analytic Review of the Literature, 1958–1979," *Group Health Journal,* Winter 1980, pp. 2–23.
18. American Medical Association, "Study of Health, Maintenance Organizations," p. 20.
19. Geisel, Jerry, "25% of HMOs Could Die of Thirst if Congress Turns Off Funding Spigot," *Modern Healthcare* (June 1981), p. 106.
20. American Medical Association, "Study of Health Maintenance Organizations," p. 125.
21. Ibid.

5

Hospital strategy in
a maturing market

It should be clear from the foregoing analysis that the hospital will be the most stressed component in a maturing health care market. How to manage the transition to a more intensely competitive economic environment, whether created by fiscal pressures or policy changes in health financing, will be the principal challenge facing hospital managers, trustees, and medical staffs. Survival in the tightening health care market will depend upon making sound strategic choices regarding the mission and structure of the hospital as well as on its relationship to its own professional staffs and to other actors in the regional market for health care.

In order to frame these strategic choices, it is useful to examine how other sectors of the U.S. economy responded to maturation of their respective markets and how these responses were reflected in the structures and strategies of individual firms and their industries. In his analysis of the changing strategies and structures of four of the nation's most successful corporations, the eminent business historian Alfred Chandler demonstrated certain underlying patterns of adaptation to market change.[1] This chapter will explore the implications of Chandler's thesis for the evolving structure of the health care industry and the place of the hospital in it.

STRUCTURAL RESPONSE TO A MATURING MARKET

In his classic study, *Strategy and Structure,* Chandler examined the changing structure of more than 100 of the nation's industrial enterprises during the late 19th and early 20th centuries. His purpose was to detect underlying principles that guided the evolution of those firms which came to dominate their respective markets. Through detailed analysis of four firms operating in widely different markets (Du Pont, General Motors, Sears, and Standard Oil of New Jersey), Chandler traced the parallel development in widely different industries of the modern, multidivisional corporation.

According to Chandler, these firms went through four distinct phases in their evolution: initial expansion and accumulation of resources; internal rationalization and consolidation of growth; diversification into new products and expansion into new markets; and, finally, development of the decentralized, multidivisional form of corporate organization. Each of these phases represented a strategic adaptation to the tightening of the market for the firm's products and to the increasing demands for coordination of the firm's internal operations. Chandler makes clear that many of these developments were defensive responses to changing competitive market conditions.

Some examples of this evolution may help to clarify the pattern. The great industrial boom in the United States was triggered by the Civil War. War driven demand stimulated the manufacturing sector of this country, which was, until the middle 1800s, largely a cottage industry. The industrial boom transformed many of these firms into large organizations. When the war ended, the nation entered into a painful period of economic readjustment, declining postwar demand, and changing trade conditions in international markets. These readjustments produced a severe depression in the 1870s and several major recessions in the 1880s and 1890s.

The maturing market for manufactured goods triggered a sequence of responses in the affected industries.

One of those responses was rapid *horizontal consolidation* of firms into larger business units. These combinations began with informal industry groupings like trade associations and cartels. The purpose of these initial attempts at industry cooperation was simple enough—to protect profit margins by preventing prices from falling. According to Chandler, these were largely ineffective because democratic means were simply unable to prevent individual actors from taking advantage of their colleagues. Responding to this problem, the more powerful economic actors in particular industries began acquiring control over their weaker competitors either by purchasing them outright or, through a variety of legal and extra-legal means, driving them out of business. Out of this raw exercise of economic power rose the trusts and holding companies which came to dominate much of U.S. industry.

In the steel industry, for example, the entrepreneur Elbert Gary, with the support of J. P. Morgan, combined the Illinois Steel and Lorain Steel Companies and Minnesota Iron Company into the Federal Steel Company. These and other consolidations led to defensive consolidations of the fabricators who needed steel, many of which in turn developed their own steel manufacturing capabilities. These developments led in turn to a billion dollar merger of the Federal, Carnegie, and National Steel Companies and many of the metal fabricating companies who bought their products, which created the United States Steel Corporation. Similar patterns of consolidation took place in other manufacturing industries.

As they struggled to survive in this tightening market, individual firms also *integrated vertically* from their manufacturing base to control more of the supply of raw materials and the distribution of their finished goods in their respective markets. In the steel industry, for example, the Carnegie Steel Company, responding to the severe economic troubles of the 1890s and the rapid consolidation of competing steel companies, purchased vast holdings of iron ore lands in the Mesabi Range of northern Minnesota near Lake Superior. The purchase was intended to assure a steady supply of low-priced ore as an alternative to continued reliance on independent ore brokers and wholesalers. Other firms followed suit. Many of these firms developed railroads and fleets of ore boats to assure prompt delivery of raw materials to their plants. This pattern of integration of the supply of raw materials is known as *backward integration*.

At the same time, many firms *integrated forward* (that is, forward toward the customer) either by buying out the wholesale distributors of their products or by developing their own sales forces and distribution networks (branch offices, warehouses, etc.). The purpose was to assure timely delivery of goods and to capture profits that would otherwise be lost to middlemen. One of the classic examples of forward integration was the development by the Swift meatpacking company of a network of refrigerated warehouses and rail cars to carry their fresh meat from Chicago packing houses to local markets. Resistance to their product by local butchers and by the railroads necessitated both active marketing of the new product and control over distribution.

In both forward and backward integration, firms applied the economies of scale of large firms to absorb profits which, in a more fragmented system, would have flowed to a network of independent economic actors. The combination of external market control and internal managerial control contributed to the economic strength of these firms, enabling them to weather difficult competitive conditions.

Chandler demonstrated that having accumulated resources and extended market control, surviving firms entered a second phase of development—rationalizing economic control over their expanded operations. This meant developing the accounting and information systems which permitted managers to exert internal control and improve productivity. In many firms, this led to the functional organization of management activities (accounting, finance, marketing, purchasing, etc.) reporting to the firm's chief executive.

Having consolidated internal managerial control, under continuing external competitive pressure the firms entered a third phase of evolution. They *diversified*, developing new products for their existing markets, and *expanded*, in many cases overseas, *into new markets.* In some cases, this was accomplished by augmenting existing product lines, and in others by acquiring firms in related businesses. Many firms set up research and development operations to uncover new technology and apply new scientific discoveries to product development. Such diversification typically led to more efficient use of existing productive capacity and was usually in product areas related to the firm's original products.

This third phase of evolution created further internal management strains which led, according to Chandler, to a fourth phase, further realignment of corporate structure. In this phase, functional organization gave way to a decentralized, multidivisional structure where corporate officers provided only general strategic and broad resource allocation guidance to operating divisions. These divisions and their managers were given considerable autonomy to manage production and control their distribution to respective markets. The separation of strategic corporate from line divisional management was the culmination of the process of evolution of these large firms. General Motors is the most widely cited example of this type of corporate organization.

Chandler's conclusion is that the firms which came to dominate their respective industries underwent a common set of strategic adaptations to the tightening market conditions. The initial period of development of resources (plant, equipment, personnel, materials and distribution system) was followed by structural change in the organization, mandated by internal control problems of the enlarged enterprise and by market pressure to lower the unit cost of goods produced.

Under continuing market pressure, firms were then compelled to a further strategic alteration in their missions— diversification into new products and new markets. The growth in scale and complexity brought about by diversification led to a further structural change, which created the modern, multidivisional corporation. According to Chandler's thesis, structural changes follow strategic adaptation to the market. Those firms which were able to adapt survived and prospered. Those which were unable to adapt failed or were absorbed by their more successful competitors. While one tends to resist using biological metaphors to describe complex human institutions, the similarity of Chandler's thesis to that of biological evolution, Darwin's "survival of the fittest," is rather striking.

RELEVANCE TO THE HEALTH CARE INDUSTRY

As discussed in the introduction, health care is not a commodity but the most intimate of personal services. Comparing the hospital to a factory is not particularly useful for a variety of reasons. However, at the level of the industry there are striking analogs in the contemporary health care market to the pattern Chandler saw in manufacturing. The market for inpatient hospital services, the most capital intensive "product" of the health care system, is maturing rapidly, and it is entering a new phase of intense market competition. Both of the structural developments Chandler identified with the initial phase of industry growth, horizontal consolidation and vertical integration, are taking place in the health care system at an accelerating rate. Approximately 30 percent of the nation's hospitals are now part of multihospital systems, a form of corporate organization that was virtually nonexistent 15 years ago.

At the same time, hospitals have been integrating vertically, developing their own distribution (feeder) networks and, in some cases, procurement systems for their scarcest resource, health professionals. Over the last 15 years, the health care industry has begun its own evolution from one of the country's last cottage industries into new forms of corporate organization which, both structurally and managerially, resemble those structures Chandler studied in the manufacturing sector of the U.S. economy.

In examining the evolution of the U.S. health care industry, Odin Anderson has divided the last 100 years into three distinct periods: development of infrastructure, development of the financing system, and rationalization of health care resources.[2]

The development of the health care infrastructure, principally the nation's hospitals, took place at an explosive pace. In 1875, there were only 175 hospitals in the United States and only 65,000 physicians for a population of 45 million.

Due to the relatively primitive state of clinical medicine, these hospitals were as much warehouses for the dying as treatment centers. However, with the development of two key medical advances, antisepsis and anaesthesia, which spurred the growth and acceptance of surgery, clinical medicine advanced rapidly.

The result was an extraordinary expansion of hospital capacity and a parallel expansion of professional personnel. By 1917 there were 5,000 hospitals and 148,000 physicians to care for a population of 103 million persons. By 1930 the number of hospitals had risen to 6,700. Much of this hospital development was stimulated by private philanthropy, the social byproduct of industrial fortunes accumulated by entrepreneurial capitalists. The growth of the voluntary hospital as a not-for-profit charitable enterprise was, according to Anderson, uniquely American.

Though private philanthropy extended beyond capital support to payment for care to the indigent, the majority of resources devoted to paying for health care were from fees from private patients. The prosperity of a rising middle class made it possible for American hospitals to support themselves through this initial phase of expansion on private patient revenues, another unique feature of the American system.

Though Anderson's period of development of infrastructure ends in 1930, an important augmentation of hospital capacity took place after World War II. The depression and the war brought conventional hospital capital development to a halt. Yet many areas and small towns lacked hospital facilities. Recognizing both the problem and the political opportunities it presented, Congress in 1946 passed the Hospital Survey and Construction Act, popularly known as the Hill-Burton Program. This program led to the addition or new construction of 340,000 hospital beds during the next 25 years, completing the development of this country's hospital infrastructure.

Anderson's second phase, ,the development of financing mechanisms, began in the early 1930s. As the complexity of hospital care and, consequently, the cost increased, a larger group of Americans, particularly of the working classes, became unable to pay the full costs of their hospital care. According to Anderson, these financial pressures stimulated the industry to develop hospital insurance plans. During the 1930s in a number of different states, hospitals sponsored Blue Cross health insurance plans under cooperative arrangements. These developments were followed closely by a parallel development of Blue Shield plans for insuring separately the cost of physicians services.

The enactment of social security in 1935 gave rise to a national debate over extending social insurance to cover health care. Owing to a variety of factors, principally the opposition of organized medicine to government involvement in financing health care, this debate continued for fully 30 years before producing the Medicare and Medicaid financing systems. With the enactment of Medicare and Medicaid, the vast majority (more than 90 percent) of hospital care became covered by private or public health insurance. By 1965, Anderson's second period of development of financing mechanisms was completed.

The third period of development in Anderson's analysis commenced in 1965 with increasing social efforts to control and rationalize health care spending. In response to this comprehensive third-party coverage of hospital care and, some speculate, the retrospective cost-based reimbursement system used by most of these payers, hospitalization costs soared. Beginning the middle 1960s, the government attempted to stimulate local control over health resources, first through Comprehensive Health Planning and subsequently through the Health Systems agencies. Neither program had a discernible impact in slowing the growth in hospital costs. By the mid-1970s, containment of hospital costs had risen to the top rank of the nation's health care policy issues.

At this stage of their evolution hospitals are being compelled by market pressures to reexamine their structures and missions as well as their management philosophy. In the Chandler pattern the hospital industry is in the middle of the first phase of industry evolution—the period of resource accumulation and market control. Some of its larger corporate actors to be discussed below are already entering the period of rationalization of resources and enhancement of productivity. Following Chandler's outline, it will be a period of "shaking out" within the industry, during which time those institutions that can develop flexible, responsive management structures and the control systems needed to render their services price competitive will consolidate their control over the hospital market.

The remainder of this book will explore the strategic issues which will be raised by the coming period of economic competition. The succeeding chapter will deal with the three principal strategic mandates facing hospitals in this changing environment. They are:

1. Horizontal consolidation of hospitals with each other into multihospital systems.
2. Vertical integration of individual and multihospital enterprises and diversification into new lines of health care delivery.
3. Realignment of relationships with the core health professionals without which the system cannot function—physicians and nurses.

Hospitals which intend to survive the coming industry shake-out are going to have to resolve problems in each of these areas and develop strategies and relationships which permit them to be competitive.

For an industry that has historically been both fragmented and managerially conservative, adjusting to these three strategic challenges facing hospitals is going to be painful and difficult. Neither hospital administrators nor physicians have, as a general rule, adapted well to the entrepreneurs in their midsts. In part this has been because, until recently, overt entrepreneurship has been viewed as neither necessary nor legitimate by either group. It is clear, however, that entrepreneurial energies must be liberated by institutions which intend to survive the tightening market for health care. Both health care management and physician practice must accommodate entrepreneurship within the administrative and professional practices, and prepare their institutions to respond with alacrity to changing economic opportunities.

NOTES

1. Alfred Chandler, *Strategy and Structure: Chapters in the History of the American Industrial Enterprise*, (Cambridge, Mass.: MIT Press, 1962).

2. Odin Anderson, "Why We Are Where We Are," University of Chicago Center for Health Administration Studies, workshop, January 29, 1981.

6 | Horizontal consolidation: The multihospital system

The traditional American hospital has been a community-based, freestanding enterprise, drawing upon local political and financial resources for its support. With the exception of a few large municipal hospital systems, such as that of New York City, most hospitals have developed in isolation from one another both clinically and managerially. But in the decade of the 1970s this fragmentation gave way to increasing interinstitutional cooperation. As we enter the 1980s, the completely freestanding hospital is rapidly becoming a thing of the past.

Over 80 percent of the nation's hospitals now participate in some form of sharing of services.[1] Approximately 30 percent are part of formal systems. As we will explore below, these systems have a wide variation in the extent of central direction and control.

Two recent surveys of multihospital systems have attempted to determine the scope and structure of multihospital cooperation. *Modern Healthcare* surveyed 176 organizations during 1980 and reported that 294,199 hospital beds in 1,681 institutions were part of a multihospital systems (Figure 6–1). Under the auspices of the American Hospital Association's Hospital Research and Education Trust, Montague Brown surveyed 245 organizations and found 301,894 beds and 1,519 institutions involved in such systems (Figure 6–2). The Brown definition of a system was somewhat broader than that of *Modern Healthcare* and incorporated affiliated institutions as well as those which were owned or managed.

Given the diversity and complexity of corporate structures, it is not surprising that estimates of the extent of multihospital cooperation vary considerably. There is no uniform typology. Both surveys understated the bed counts of hospitals owned or operated by investor owned hospital management companies during 1979. Nevertheless, the surveys appear to establish that about 30 percent of the nation's hospital beds are part of multihospital systems as of 1979. Multihospital organization may range from informal cooperative arrangements to formal corporate ownership and control.

Figure 6–3 illustrates the spectrum of possible organizational arrangements along with key features relating to governance and control. The key to the efficiency of holding companies and consolidated models is the centralization of budgeting and financial controls and the allocation of capital on a system wide basis. As Brown points out, the further to the right one moves on Figure 6–3, the less policymaking autonomy is accorded the chief executive officer of the hospital, and the less control is likely to be exerted by the hospital's medical staff over resource allocation.

Montague Brown also made a useful attempt at distinguishing the gross numbers and characteristics of systems according to the degree of centralization of management. Under managed systems, Brown distinguished between those hospitals managed directly from a corporate office and those managed on a decentralized basis with some autonomy accorded the hospital chief executive officer (CEO). These managed systems include the investor owned hospital management companies. Brown also identified systems in which hospitals were not managed from or through a corporate office but participated as affiliates. This affiliated systems

FIGURE 6–1
Total beds and units

Type of system	Total beds owned/leased and managed			Total units owned/leased and managed			Systems reporting		
	change	1980	1979	change	1980	1979	change	1980	1979
Religious	+4.4%	110,740	106,062	+8.1%	492	455	+1.5%	69	68
Investor owned	+14.0%	103,280	90,580	+15.4%	802	695	+3.0%	34	33
Secular nonprofit	+4.1%	58,731	56,398	+9.3%	329	301	+1.8%	58	57
Public	−1.2%	21,448	21,718	−1.7%	58	59	0	15	15
Total	+7.1%	294,199	274,758	+11.3%	1,681	1,510	+1.8%	176	173

Source: Reprinted from the April, 1981 issue of *Modern Healthcare,* copyright, Crain Communications, Inc., all rights reserved.

FIGURE 6–2
Multihospital systems by type of ownership

	Number of systems	Percent of total	Number of beds	Percent of total
Investor owned.......	27	11%	63,477	21%
Catholic	123	50%	139,974	46%
Other religious	29	11%	27,666	9%
Voluntary	44	17%	37,796	13%
Medical center	7	2%	8,141	3%
Government	15	6%	24,840	8%
Total	245	100%	301,894	100%

Source: Reprinted by permission, Montague Brown, "Multihospital Systems: Trends, Issues, Prospects," HRET Invitational Conference on Multihospital Systems, March 18, 1980, p. 5.

category was further broken down to reflect the degree of input the coordinating body had in selecting the hospital CEO.

It can be seen in Figure 6–4 that the decentralized managed systems have the largest number of beds per system, reflecting the enhanced ability of a decentralized organization to manage a larger number of units. In comparing growth rates from an earlier survey conducted in 1975 Brown concluded that, for those systems surveyed both times, the affiliated systems shrank slightly over four years while the managed systems grew substantially, both in numbers of beds and numbers of hospitals. Considered in the context of the spectrum of control represented in the Montague Brown typology, the growth is occurring on the holding company end of the spectrum, whether in investor owned firms or regional nonprofit settings.

HOSPITAL MANAGEMENT FIRMS

In 1980, investor owned hospital management companies owned or operated (under management contract) 862 of the nation's nonfederal acute hospitals, or 12.3 percent of the hospital market. These hospitals contained a total of 108,048 beds. The number of hospitals controlled by these firms grew by 80 percent from 1975 to 1980. Investor owned hospitals, both independent and multiunit, accounted for 18.1 percent of the nation's hospitals in 1979. Independent investor owned

FIGURE 6-3
Control and impact by type of system

	Single hospital	Program affiliation	Shared service organization	Contract management	Consortia	Condominium	Holding company	Total consolidation
Actors involved								
Board	X	As appropriate			X	X	X	X
Medical staff	X	X		X	X	X	Varies	Varies
Administration	X	As appropriate			X	X	Varies	Varies
Hospital department	X		X	X	X	X	X	X
Resource allocation control								
Primarily local	X	X			X	X		
Joint over program		X	X	X	X	X		
Central for capital							X	X
Central for operations							X	X
Joint for common areas						X		X
Governing structure	Board	Committee	Varies	Board	Joint board	Joint board	Multiple boards	Single board
Medical staff organizations	Single	Single	Single	Single	Coordination	Varies	Varies	Varies
CEO autonomy								
Policy	High	High	High	Medium	High	Medium	Medium	Low
Operations	High	High	High	High	High	High	High	High

Source: Reprinted from *Multihospital Systems Strategies for Organization and Management* by Montague Brown and Barbara McCool, by permission of Aspen Systems Corp., © 1980.

FIGURE 6–4
Change in selected characteristics of 200 systems surveyed (1975 and 1979)

	Managed		Affiliated		Total
	Centralized	Decentralized	Coordinated	Autonomous	
Number of systems	28	74	78	22	202
Percent of total	13%	36%	38%	10%	100%
Beds per system:					
1975	931	1586	952	863	1140
1979	1064	1982	947	851	1332
Percent increase	14%	25%	−1%	−1%	17%
Hospitals per system:					
1975	5.3	8.8	4.0	3.5	5.9
1979	6.6	10.9	3.9	3.1	6.8
Percent increase	24%	24%	−2%	−11%	15%
Beds per hospital:					
1975	175	181	237	243	195
1979	161	182	240	271	197
Percent increase	−8%	1%	1%	12%	1%

Source: Montague Brown, "Multihospital Systems: Trends, Issues, Prospects," HRET Invitational Conference on Multihospital Systems, March 18, 1980, p. 17.

hospitals, which are generally physician owned, account for a shrinking proportion of investor owned hospitals. Hospital management firms accounted for 41.1 percent of all investor owned facilities in 1975 and for 63.8 percent of such facilities in 1980.[2] If the present rate of growth of market share by hospital management firms continues at its present pace in the next five years, they will control more than 1,500 hospitals in 1985, more than one fifth of all hospitals in the country (that is, nonfederal acute care "community" hospitals).

While 38 companies were involved in hospital management in 1980, over 61 percent of the market is controlled by five large organizations—Hospital Corporation of America, Hospital Affiliates International (a division of INA Corporation since acquired by HCA), Humana, American Medical International, and National Medical Enterprises. The largest of these companies, Hospital Corporation of America, expected to control approximately 200 hospitals by the end of its 1980–81 fiscal year, but after its acquisition of Hospital Affiliates, controlled 345 hospitals and nearly 43,000 beds.

Investor owned hospitals are not evenly distributed geographically and the hospital management firms mirror this distribution. Hospitals in the Northeast and upper Midwest account for only about 12 percent of all investor owned facilities. In contrast, 58 percent of all investor owned hospitals are located in five states—California, Texas, Florida, Tennessee, and New York. The management firms have concentrated their acquisitions and contracts in the sunbelt states. Their degree of penetration of investor-owned markets in these states is extremely high—ranging from 63 percent of all investor-owned hospital beds in the state of California to almost 85 percent of all investor owned beds in Tennessee.

These states have a number of features in common—a favorable climate of health regulation, Blue Cross plans which pay generous hospital benefits (usually at the level of charges), and relatively low labor costs (reflecting a low level of unionization of the hospital work force). The firms have thus far avoided states with punititive hospital rate review systems or strong Certificate of Need laws. Western and midwestern states should anticipate increased market presence of these firms as the relatively lucrative southern and border state markets already tapped begin to saturate.

There are several areas of significant market potential for hospital management firms in the future. The latter part of the 1970s saw increasing growth in management contracting among these firms. In 1980 the firms had 342 hospitals under contract, representing 36,798 beds. This represents a 13 percent increase in hospitals and a 14 percent increase in beds under management contract in only one year. Management companies operated approximately 69 percent of the 493 hospitals under management contracts in 1980, the remaining operating being nonprofit organizations of various types.[3]

The most rapid growth occurred in municipal and county owned facilities. Fully one third of the facilities under contract are municipal or county owned.[4] This segment of the market has significant growth potential as financially pressed local governments* seek management expertise in operating increasingly expensive municipal public hospitals. The most visible movement in this sector came in 1979 when Hyatt Medical Corporation, now a division of American Medical International, signed a three-year contract to manage the troubled 1,300-bed Cook County Hospital in Chicago. Since there are about 1,900 public/general hospitals in the country, the market potential in this sector appears to be very high for further penetration by contract management and perhaps ultimately by ownership.

Contract management is, financially, a low-risk proposition for the hospital management firms and their nonprofit competitors. It provides firms a low cost method of assessing the profit potential of a hospital and the tractibility of local and regional labor markets and regulatory systems. Contract management frequently provides preferential access to future purchase of the facility as well as potentially large discounts in the purchase prices. Though the management firms have an edge in the contract management field, their nonprofit system competitors have doubled their share of the market in 1979 as compared to 1978 and continued rapid growth in 1980, as can be seen in figure 6–5.

---

* Many of these government units are local hospital taxing districts in rural areas which were created to take advantage of Hill Burton grants.

FIGURE 6-5
Contract management summary

Type of manager	Beds managed			Units managed			Percent share of managed beds		change	Number of managers	
	change	1980	1979	change	1980	1979	1980	1979		1980	1979
Investor-owned.......	+13.0%	36,798	32,580	+14.0%	342	300	73.3	74.1	+ 4.3%	24	23
Secular nonprofit.......	+26.3%	7,102	5,623	+37.5%	77	56	14.2	12.8	+20.0%	18	15
Religious	+ 8.7%	6,169	5,673	+12.5%	72	64	12.3	12.9	+ 8.3%	26	24
Public...............	0	99	99	0	2	2	.2	.2	0	1	1
Total......	+14.1%	50,168	43,975	+16.8%	493	422	100	100	+ 9.5%	69	63

Source: Reprinted from the April, 1981 issue of *Modern Healthcare*, copyright, Crain Communications, Inc., all rights reserved.

Recently the Health Care Financing Administration (HCFA) has begun moving to restrict the profitability of management contracting by subjecting management fees to "reasonable cost" review. The balance of growth between contract management and ownership by hospital management firms could shift back in the direction of ownership if the HCFA efforts succeed. In the meantime the large firms, and their nonprofit system competitors, have sensed the major market opportunities afforded by contract management and considerable growth in this business is likely.

Another avenue of expansion of the hospital management firms is overseas. Management firms own, operate, or are constructing more than 5,500 beds in 46 hospitals abroad. Australia and England are the largest areas of current activity, though several firms have signed lucrative contracts to develop and operate facilities in Saudi Arabia.[5]

THE INVESTOR OWNED HOSPITAL CONTROVERSY

The expanding market presence of the hospital management firms has revived a public controversy over the proprietary role in a traditionally nonprofit industry. Investor owned hospitals constituted more than one third (36 percent) of the industry in 1928, when 2,435 of the nation's hospitals were investor owned.[6] This presence shrank to 769 hospitals in 1968 but has nearly doubled in the last 12 years, owing largely to the growth of management firms. Parallel growth in large corporate firm penetration has occurred in other sectors of the health care industry, including nursing homes, dialysis, and home health care.

In a controversial article in the *New England Journal of Medicine* in the fall of 1980 its editor, Dr. Arnold Relman, wrote of the threat of this new "medical industrial complex" to the legitimacy of the medical profession and to its objectivity in the debate over national health policy.[7] He urged that physicians separate themselves from ownership or financial involvement in health care enterprises and called for increased regulation of for-profit providers of health care.

In a less visible but equally important essay, Robert Clark, a professor of law at Harvard, took an opposite tack. He examined the premises of the "social charter" granted to the nonprofit hospitals (for example, favored tax treatment) and concluded that nonprofit hospitals are less likely to be efficient. Clark argued that nonprofit hospitals were not returning benefits to society commensurate with their protection and recommended abolishing the legal and regulatory distinctions between for-profit and not-for-profit hospitals.[8]

The charge most often leveled at the management firms is that they "skim the cream" from local markets. That is, because the firms have a profit objective, they will tilt the hospital's programs away from money losing services (obstetrics, for example) or restrict access to service of public assistance recipients. These charges are extremely difficult to document and have yet to be supported by a single reputable published research study. However, many nonprofit hospitals which moved from inner city to suburban locations in the 1950s and 1960s did so to avoid the increasing burden of caring for the indigent. The extent to which the large firms engage in this practice may vary from firm to firm.

Another point of controversy is absentee ownership and management of local facilities. Most firms have found it important to retain local boards for the hospitals and invest in community and public relations to tell the firm's story. Some of the benefits of firm entry into local markets are apt to be overlooked by local residents, but they frequently include assistance in recruiting physicians and nurses into rural and small town settings, outside capital funding of renovations or replacement of local facilities, and relief of local tax burdens through reduction in operating deficits of publicly owned facilities.

Yet another area of controversy concerns the relative cost of care in proprietary facilities. A 1978 study of the cost of care by Lewin and Associates showed significantly higher costs for proprietary hospitals than comparable non-profit hospitals.* This study was criticized by the management firms on methodological grounds. Subsequent research conducted by Carson Bays answered part of the criticism of

---

* This finding was echoed by a second Lewin study sponsored by a group of non-profit multihospital systems. This 1980 study found that while the investor owned hospitals had only slightly higher costs, they "priced their services considerably higher above costs, resulting in higher profits." See Lewin, Derzon, and Margulies, *Hospitals,* July 1, 1981, p. 32.

the Lewin Study by correcting the costs of sample hospitals by case mix—that is, correcting for the relative seriousness of illness in hospitals according to patient diagnosis. The Bays study, published in 1979, concluded:

> For-profits as a group appear to be significantly less costly than non-profits after accounting for differences in case mix. . . . Moreover, chain for-profit hospitals—those which are part of broadly owned hospital corporations—have case loads which are not significantly different from those of non-profits, but appear to be less costly than non-profits and non-chain for-profits as well.[9]

Bays attributed the latter finding to possible economies of scale in the large hospital management firms.

More recent research has confirmed the Bays findings. Using a sample of 2,800 hospitals over a 10-year period (1970–79), researchers at ABT Associates established that cost per adjusted patient admission rose by 1 percent less in proprietary hospitals than in nonprofits over the period.[10]

The management firms have several advantages over free-standing or nonprofit competitors. The most significant is access to capital. The larger management firms have access to the equity markets and are listed on the New York Stock Exchange. Hospital management firms have been among the hottest groups in a troubled stock market over the last five years and have experienced significant earnings growth and concommitant appreciation in the value of their shares.

Access to equity markets provides these firms the means to fuel further expansion. In addition, their aftertax cash flows, while not massive as a percentage of gross revenues, still represent a nondebt source of capital financing and the basis as well for access to commercial bonds at favorable interest rates.* Finally, in many states these firms have access to debt markets through industrial revenue bonds. Even

---

* Medicare reimbursement provides for-profit hospitals a financial edge over nonprofits by permitting a 2 percent return on equity factor to be incorporated into the hospital cost base. This has certainly benefited for-profit hospitals and firms who concentrated their activity among communities with large elderly populations. Precise estimates of the additional cash flows are not readily available.

though nonprofits have access to tax-exempt bond markets at highly favorable rates, access to capital is likely to remain the biggest edge the hospital management firms have over their nonprofit competitors.

Second, many firms have already penetrated international markets. As domestic market pressures mount the larger firms will also be positioned to increase net income from their foreign operations, where they can operate almost completely free from regulatory (though not from political) constraints. These foreign cash flows can be used to subsidize continued domestic expansion or diversification into other health care product lines. Hospital Corporation of America puts the potential size of this foreign market at $500 billion annually,[11] more than double the size of the domestic market. Hospital Corporation of America has taken advantage of its foreign market presence to alleviate the nursing shortage in its hospitals by recruiting nurses from abroad. Thus the large firms may be positioned both to export American health management expertise and technology and to import personnel in shortage areas. This international reach can provide significant resources to bring to bear on increasingly tight domestic markets.

Management technology is a third area where the large firms in particular seem to have a competitive edge. Centralized computing systems keyed to sophisticated management software (for accounting, cost reimbursement, inventory, and position control) and highly developed productivity standards for each major hospital cost center help these firms increase operational efficiency and net revenues after a hospital has been acquired. The two problems most frequently cited in acquired hospitals are overstaffing in nursing and support personnel and failure to maximize cost reimbursement. Correcting these problems frequently yields major savings and increased revenues. These system approaches are not necessarily restricted to the management firms but their relative size makes it possible to develop the top quality managerial and systems expertise needed.

A fourth area where the economies of scale of large firms may produce a competitive edge over nonprofits is in dealing with large suppliers. The hospital supply industry will be pressed by increasing concentration of buying power among the large firms to offer substantial discounts and favorably financial treatment to them. While group purchasing is a widespread practice in the industry already, hospital management firms may soon reach the size that the threat of acquisition or direct entry into the supply market is sufficiently credible to tilt the price of hospital supplies in their favor.

Hospital management firms have been criticized for concentrating on acquiring isolated small hospitals in relatively secure local markets. The implication is that the small hospital is easier to manage. The investor owned firms are sensitive to this criticism and point out that the average size of their facilities is greater than the average size of independent proprietaries. However, the average size of the facilities managed by these firms was only 125 beds,[12] compared to a national average for community hospitals of 168 beds.[13]

The firms have had the flexibility to add or drop hospitals from their portfolios according to their assessment of the hospital's potential profitability. Some critics have suggested that at this stage of their evolution the firms are really managing portfolios of properties rather than hospitals. The term *marketing* in many of these organizations, unfortunately, is still synonymous with *acquisitions*. As firms reach the point of saturating local markets, as is happening rapidly in such areas as Houston and Nashville, the firms will be pressed into direct competition with one another and with regionally based systems in metropolitan areas, and the name of the game will change.

In the evolutionary scheme of Alfred Chandler these firms, some of which are growing at 20 to 30 percent annual rates, are well advanced into the second phase of corporate evolution—rationalization of the use of resources. They have well-developed capital structures, information and control systems, and productivity standards. These features will enable the firms to compete vigorously and successfully in price-conscious markets while moving to consolidate control over them. Following Chandler, however, at the point where saturation of profitable sunbelt and border state markets is reached, the firms will be pressed to grow in two directions—

diversification into other forms of health care and expansion into other domestic and foreign markets.

Several of the larger firms, notably National Medical Enterprises and Hospital Affiliates International, have taken major positions in nursing home management, for example. Other firms, such as Hospital Corporation of America have, at least thus far, eschewed new product development, concentrating their strategy on building as large a base of hospitals as possible. At the same time, however, through its unique research and development subsidiary, The Center for Health Studies, HCA is experimenting with new forms of care such as primary care centers and surgicenters linked to their hospitals, for possible addition to their facilities in the future.

Still others, such as the Hyatt Medical Corporation, now a division of American Medical International, have staked out a strong position in the largest domestic market segment through contract management of municipal and county hospitals. Through its long-standing contract relationship with the Tulane Medical Center Hospitals and Clinics, Hospital Affiliates is staking out its position in a more specialized and troublesome teaching hospital segment.

At this point it is difficult to speculate about the outer limits of growth of these firms, though it is conceivable that they could eventually control as many as one half of the nation's hospitals and a comparable portion of the nation's nursing homes. Some highly regulated markets in the United States, particularly in the Northeast and upper Midwest, may remain so unattractive that the firms will avoid these areas, though low-risk contract management remains an option here. At some point, however, it will no longer be practical, either for reasons of unattractive opportunities or perhaps span of control and coordination problems, to grow at anything approaching recent rates.

When this point is reached the firms will face the fourth stage of Chandler's evolution—development of new structures for managing the expanded, diversified base. To expand and hold market shares in particular metropolitan areas or substate regions will require formal marketing strategies keyed to each area. The period of rapid growth of these firms will inevitably be followed by a period of consolidation and knitting together of facilities and services at the local level. These strategies will key the recruitment and retention of medical staff, the development of formal linkages between the clinical services of firms' regional hospitals and development of vertically integrated health care linkages encompassing ambulatory care and aftercare services, and the relationships to competing health plans in the region.

Management at this scale and detail will be literally impossible from a national corporate office or even from large, multistate regional offices. These pressures for fine-tuning local markets will eventually compel the firms to manage by metropolitan area or by substate region, since these are generally the outer geographic limits of most health care markets. Per Chandler's corporate model, local system managers will be given considerable operational autonomy in achieving and holding their market position. The ultimate battle for control over the health care market will be at the local level since there is no national market for health services.

Despite the uncertainties of future regulatory and market conditions, the future of the hospital management firms appears to be very bright indeed. How far these firms will penetrate into the inner city and into heavily regulated markets before pushing more aggressively abroad will be interesting to watch. Yet these firms have brought a philosophy of corporate management and accountability to the field which will galvanize not-for-profit competitors to organize themselves to compete.

REGIONAL NONPROFIT SYSTEMS

While a lot of national attention is focused on the hospital management firms, it is easy to overlook the fact that the nonprofit multihospital systems outnumber the management firms on every dimension—units owned or managed, beds, and assets.

According to *Modern Healthcare's* 1979 survey, nonprofit systems added beds at a 12 percent rate compared to 1978 and the Protestant systems at a 22 percent rate, compared to a 7 percent rate for the investor owned systems. During 1980 the investor owned systems grew by 14 percent compared to around 4 percent of secular and religious systems.[14] With one significant exception, the Kaiser Permanente Medical Care Program (the largest nonprofit health system in the United States with 6,235 beds in 29 Kaiser hospitals), these systems are regionally based, generally spanning no more than two or at most three states. The largest of these systems are organized, implicitly or explicitly, around religious denominations. After Kaiser, the 11 largest are Catholic systems (the largest being the Sisters of Mercy Health Corporation of Farmington Hills, Michigan, which operates 22 hospitals with 5,461 beds in Michigan, Iowa, and Indiana). Approximately 43 percent of the 640 Catholic hospitals in the country were listed by *Modern Healthcare* as being a part of a multihospital system.[15] Ninety percent of the Catholic hospitals in the country are sponsored by religious congregations, the remainder by dioceses or lay groups.[16]

The Adventist hospitals in the United States have recently reorganized into four strong, regionally based systems, and seem to be moving cautiously toward some national planning and possible consolidation.[17] Three of the four largest Protestant hospital systems in the country (ranging in size from 2,446 to 2,712 beds in 1979) are Adventist systems. The Lutherans have two very large hospital systems, one based in southern California and the other in Fargo, North Dakota. In all of these cases, the health care mission of these systems is seen as an extension of the church's ministry. Varying degrees of accountability to church leadership, both locally and nationally, are implied in these organizations. Published data on the extent to which these systems provide financial support for the religious orders and congregations which sponsor them are difficult to obtain. In some cases, however, the scale of hospital operations has dwarfed the religious order, creating nervousness among church leadership and sowing the seeds of possible governance problems in the future.

Many of the secular nonprofit systems in the country were built around wealthy, successful core teaching hospitals. The Samaritan Health Service was built around the 700-bed Good

Samaritan Hospital of Phoenix. Henry Ford Hospital of Detroit and Presbyterian-St. Lukes Hospital and Medical Center in Chicago have both spawned large multihospital systems. One of the larger Protestant multihospital systems in the country, the Evangelical Hospital Association of Oak Brook, Illinois, was built around its successful suburban giant, the 830-bed Christ Hospital.

This latter system's evolution is particularly interesting. Stung by criticism from the community and from its own religious order for withdrawing from its original inner city location, the Evangelical Hospital Association moved back into the inner city in the late 1970s by acquiring two troubled community hospitals on Chicago's south and west sides. Suburban profits are thus being channelled back into the inner city to areas which are critically short of both hospital facilities and physicians.

These systems built around core hospitals face the problem of how to manage the inevitable relations of subsidy between the core facility and the frequently costly new ventures. Large hospitals are capital-hungry enterprises. It is difficult to manage capital resources on a system-wide basis if the medical staff of the core facility believes its resources are being diverted to serve the needs of other physicians.

Most of the large multihospital systems develop a corporate office to handle system-wide planning; budgeting, including capital; key personnel (CEOs); interfaces with key government agencies; and whatever centralized services (group purchasing, computer system, etc.) the system may commit to providing. Varying degrees of autonomy for operating the constituent hospitals of the system are delegated to the chief executive officers of system hospitals. There is inevitable tension between "corporate" and the operating officers in such systems, an outgrowth of an additional layer of constraints upon complete exercise of management responsibility. Some of these systems also experience difficulty recruiting chief executive officers for their larger institutions because such individuals are given titles like vice president, when in freestanding organizations they would be presidents of their organizations with a direct reporting relationship to the board of trustees.

Though health planners have enthusiastically encouraged the development of multihospital systems to promote cost containment, there has yet to be any conclusive evidence that these systems actually save money. In fact, the staff and costs associated with development of a new layer of corporate management, and with starting up such new ventures as joint purchasing, may actually increase system costs in the short run.

Unlike the hospital management firms, which have invested considerable resources in the last 10 years to develop management control systems, the new multihospital systems must frequently develop this expertise from scratch. And because of the history of past autonomy on the part of system hospitals, there may be resistance to developing the type of detailed financial accountability demanded by the large hospital management firms. Nevertheless, there is anecdotal evidence that well-established, nonprofit, multihospital systems can develop sufficient controls to restrain their costs below regional nonprofit competitors.

THE COMPETITIVE OUTLOOK FOR REGIONAL NON-PROFIT SYSTEMS

Because they are regional, these systems have some advantages over the national hospital management firms in competing for local contracts and possible acquisitions. First, they can claim to be part of the local community and characterize the national firms as being disinterested in the needs of local residents. Second, through their boards of trustees and medical staffs they are likely to build upon a base of local political power, which may benefit them in regulatory interactions surrounding the possible acquisition or contract, as well as in generating favorable publicity about their activities. In some cases, the medical staffs of the outlying institutions may have trained at the core hospital and have collegial ties to the medical staffs at the hospital where they trained.

Some of the larger regional nonprofits have capitalized on these local strengths to dominate their local markets. Founded in 1975, the Intermountain Health Service built upon a base of institutions formerly operated by the Mormon Church in Utah and branched into Idaho and Wyoming through management contracting and leases. It has a very strong financial position and under the aggressive leadership of its president, Scott Parker, has begun developing active referral ties between its 23-member institutions as well as a shared services network which reaches more than 50 institutions in a 6-state region. Intermountain also catalyzed the development of a captive insurance company, MultiHospital Mutual Insurance, Ltd., which insures some 72 hospitals in the region. Intermountain's position in this market is sufficiently well entrenched that it may be impossible for the management firms to dislodge it.

As mentioned above, many of the regional nonprofit systems have entered the contract management field. In some cases, this activity is conducted from the corporate office of the system. In others, it is spun off as a subsidiary corporation. Regional nonprofits view contract management as a new revenue source for the system as well as a way of extending the "reach" of their system in particular markets. Those regional systems built around a large core hospital may be looking for markets for the specialized diagnostic and treatment services of the core hospital in constituents of their system.

Since many core hospitals have extensive residency training programs or are principal teaching hospitals of medical schools, joining a regional system may be a way for a small community-based hospital to attract medical staff. Regional systems also present the possibility of developing clinical cooperation between hospitals. The national management firms have been criticized for being so horizontal that this type of cooperation between hospitals is precluded. However, just as there has been a real shortage of evidence of operating savings from development of regional systems, there has also been a shortage of evidence that this type of cooperation between medical staffs of constituent institutions of multihospital systems has in fact taken place, resulting in reduced duplication of services and, hence, reduced costs.

In some cases, the medical staffs of outlying hospitals may be overtly hostile to and competitive with the staff of the core hospital and refuse to refer patients to the core hospital for fear that the patient will be stolen. If the competitive climate in outlying communities is sufficiently intense, administrators of satellite facilities may be unable to retain their staffs without duplicating expensive clinical facilities of the core hospital (catherization laboratories, CAT scanners, etc.), vitiating the possibility of achieving system-wide economies. It may be that a more restrictive reimbursement climate, or increased economic competition may compel greater system-wide use of core tertiary-level medical facilities. The existence of a corporate superstructure may make it easier to develop clinical collaboration between hospitals within the system though system planners try to avoid imposing such patterns.

The regional systems are, as mentioned earlier, at some disadvantage over their national competitors in the ability to raise capital. In earlier years, the principal source of capital for nonprofit institutions was philanthropy. While there may be a philanthropic constituency for a successful established hospital in a community, that constituency is unlikely to generalize to the system. Thus, nonprofits are generally limited to use of retained earnings and to tax-exempt debt markets (and the implicit debt capacity of the combined hospital operations) for capital resources. While effective management can expand the debt capacity of the hospitals in the system by generating sustained net income, there is a limit to the leverage which these systems can exert. On the earnings side, recent surveys concluded that well-established regional firms have been able to generate net incomes and returns on assets which rival those of the management firms on a percentage basis.[18] However, because of the smaller revenue base of the regional nonprofits, retained earnings alone will not produce sufficient revenues to meet future capital needs.

This limited financial capacity will severely restrict systems in their ability to *purchase* additional hospitals, perhaps suggesting why they have so aggressively expanded their activity in contract management. Many nonprofit systems have been able to acquire hospitals voluntarily through mergers because the acquired hospitals have exhausted their capital resources and face major renovation or replacement of their facilities. But if these hospitals are not able to return cash flow in sufficient amounts to repay the investment, the acquisition of a hospital "for free" may not be a sound business decision.

For these reasons, it will require unusual entrepreneurial ability and, in particular, the ability to generate substantial cash flows outside the conventional hospital reimbursement for inpatient services to permit these nonprofit systems to grow. Whether religious orders will be able to subsidize their hospital systems from their own philanthropic base seems doubtful. Regional systems may resort to unbundling, a strategy which will be explored below, to generate streams of income to support additional acquisitions or diversification. Solving the problem of access to capital will be the single largest challenge facing the nonprofit systems during the 1980s.

Some creative approaches to capital financing are emerging as hospitals form consortia to pool their assets and earnings capacity to obtain larger amounts of financing at more favorable rates. These consortia stop considerably short of corporate merger and yet permit capital leverage unavailable to isolated facilities. Tax-exempt hospital bonding authorities generally permit higher debt ratios to not-for-profits than commercial lenders permit their for-profit management firm clientel. However, policy developments to restrict hospital access to tax-exempt markets or to abolish tax-exempt debt for hospitals outright could deal a fatal blow to the further development of regional nonprofit hospital systems and to nonprofit hospitals generally.

With the benefits of cost and potential clinical cooperation in doubt, one can reasonably ask why these systems are formed in the first place. Montague Brown, who has been in the forefront of studying this movement, has a possible answer when he points out that

> very little information exists which addresses most of the questions which one might logically ask in order to determine whether or not to favor the growth or development of multi-hospital systems. Those who have developed systems seem firmly convinced that they offer advantages worth pursuing. But one of the key advantages of systems has little to do directly with improved care or superior cost performance. Simply put, systems feel they

have more power, talent, resources and opportunities to influence their destinies in an increasingly competitive, regulated and politicized world.[19]

To the extent that these systems can mobilize political and managerial resources to meet changing regulatory and political conditions, they may yield dividends which are difficult to quantify. Many systems also serve other ends than direct service delivery, such as the training of health manpower. Multihospital systems may be the way in which the nonprofit hospital industry plans for its own future in regional markets, whatever the planning priorities of regulators and reimbursers of care. For this reason, because this course represents the exercise of private power in the best American tradition, it is unlikely to be merely a passing fancy in an increasingly complex industry. The survival of regional nonprofit systems in a highly competitive health care market, however, will depend upon moving from politics and planning into the aggressive corporate management mode which only a few of these systems have yet been able to achieve.

OTHER TYPES OF HORIZONTAL CONSOLIDATION

Joint ownership or management does not exhaust the possible methods of horizontal consolidation. As pointed out earlier, many of the multihospital systems in existence today do not rely on management, centralized or decentralized, to achieve joint cooperation. Many of the multihospital systems in the country are knit together by affiliations. As Brown points out in his typology, hospitals in these systems or networks get very little if any direction from the corporate office. Many of these systems are organized around academic health centers and are organized to provide services related to medical education in the community hospital setting. We will explore this type of system further in our discussion of vertically integrated systems.

There are other types of sharing which involve neither affiliation nor management. These include consortia and shared service agreements between neighboring institutions. The scope of cooperation may range from formal agreements to informal sharing, but it typically does not involve the creation of a separate administrative entity to manage the sharing. An American Hospital Association survey found that the number of nonfederal hospitals engaged in shared services grew from 61 percent in 1975 to about 82 percent in 1978.[20] The most common form of shared service was purchasing, with 77 percent of the community based institutions surveyed participating in some form of joint purchasing. Over 40 percent participated in shared data processing systems, while approximately one fourth participated in shared laundry services. There was less evidence of shared clinical services, though 36 percent of the community hospitals participating reported sharing blood bank services, 32 percent laboratory/pathology services, and 26 percent radiology services. These data suggest that it is easier to achieve interinstitutional cooperation through the administrative line in the hospital matrix than through the clinical line.

Cooperative systems may be initiated by institutions that are not satisfied with their in-house capability to provide such services and where larger joint programs sponsored by local hospital councils may not be available. They may also be initiated by institutions to share excess capacity or to exploit special managerial talent or relationships with suppliers to extend savings to other institutions. To the extent that these arrangements actually generate net income however, the flow of "unrelated business income," unless properly segregated, can result in a residual income tax liability for the nonprofit hospital.

In some circumstances, the consortium concept may extend to the provision of clinical services. Hospitals are encouraged by the Health Planning Act to develop multihospital agreements to share certain high technology services, such as CAT scanners, linear accelerators, and the like. Hospitals which have such technology may elect to market these services aggressively in the community, again with the objective of increasing their revenues as well as making their services more broadly available. Access is generally guaranteed by referral agreements.

An unusual example of the application of the consortium concept to ambulatory care services was the creation during the 1970s of a consortium to provide ambulatory services for five inner city hospitals in Detroit under the umbrella of the Medical School at Wayne State University. At the behest of the Michigan legislature, these institutions collaborated in developing a freestanding $45 million ambulatory facility, the Health Care Institute, with a capacity of 600,000 outpatient visits annually. The institute was to assume the ambulatory care responsibilities for the five hospitals, including the Detroit Municipal Hospital. Owing to inadequate planning and unrealistic assumptions about altering the practice patterns of physicians at the participating institutions, severe fiscal difficulties for the city of Detroit and Wayne County, and a host of other factors, the program foundered shortly after it was opened and is in the process of being reorganized. The strategic error in planning the facility was in trying to force well-established private practice and university-based physicians into a very large institutional practice setting. Because the effort was stimulated not by perceived physician interest but by policymakers and planners far removed from the realities of clinical practice, it has been the most spectacular failure in the relatively brief history of multihospital clinical collaboration and demonstrates that multi-institutional cooperation, while elegant conceptually, is risky and frequently very difficult to bring about.

Observers in the field generally agree that it is very difficult to achieve changes in costs or medical practice patterns on any scale if the agents of change do not formally control the budgets and personnel of the involved institutions. Even where such control exists, of course, no managerial actors control the behavior of the physician, who holds the key to a hospital's viability. Affiliations and consortia are less threatening to physicians than the creation of large corporate superstructures remote from day-to-day operation of the facility.

The rapid development of multihospital arrangements, under both proprietary and not-for-profit management, was perhaps the most striking organizational change in the hospital industry in the 1970s. It is reasonable to speculate that the number of hospitals participating in some form of system will continue to grow to the point where only a small minority of institutions remain freestanding by the end of this decade. This consolidation seems certain to raise antitrust issues as systems move to consolidate control over local markets.

However, it is difficult to speculate at this juncture about what degree of market penetration will trigger effective litigation. While the government's role in antitrust activity in health care may be muted by the Reagan administration, it will remain a potential weapon for private litigants.

Multi-hospital structures are as complex managerially as the constituent hospitals are internally. Those systems which can harnass the clinical and managerial resources of their constituent institutions, and develop the capital to diversify and expand into new health care products and markets, will eventually dominate the U.S. health care industry. The evolution of formal corporate strategy in this multihospital field (even in the management firms) is in a primitive state relative to other sectors of the U.S. industrial system. But market pressures will compel these organizations to integrate their resources and establish a corporate strategic management philosophy in hospitals which have, to date, been administered rather than truly managed.

NOTES

1. Elworth Taylor, "Survey Shows Who is Sharing Which Services," *Hospitals*, September 19, 1979.
2. Federation of American Hospitals, *1981 Directory of Investor Owned Hospitals and Hospital Management Companies* (Washington, D.C.: Federation of American Hospitals).
3. "1981 Multi-Hospital System Survey," *Modern Healthcare*, April 1981, p. 80.
4. "City, County Contracts Lead To Hospital Sales," *Modern Healthcare*, September 1980, p. 44.
5. Federation of American Hospitals, 1981 Directory.
6. Arnold Relman, "The New Medical-Industrial Complex," *New England Journal of Medicine*, October 23, 1980, p. 963.
7. Ibid.
8. Robert Clark, "Does the Non-Profit Form Fit the Hospital Industry?" *Harvard Law Review*, May 1980, p. 1,417.
9. Carson Bays, "Cost Comparisons of For-Profit and Non-Profit Hospitals," *Social Science and Medicine* 13C (December 1979), p. 224.
10. Craig Coelen and Daniel Sullivan, "An Analysis of the Effects of Prospective Reimbursement Programs on Hospital Expenditures," *Health Care Financing Review*, Winter 1981, p. 1.
11. Hospital Coropration of American, *1980 Annual Report*.
12. Federation of American Hospitals, "1979–1980 Directory—Investor Owned Hospitals and Hospital Management Companies" (Washington, D.C.: Federation of American Hospitals, 1980), pp. 11–12.
13. American Hospital Association, "Guide to the Health Care Field."

14. Donald E. L. Johnson, ed., "Multi-Hospital System Survey," *Modern Healthcare,* April 1979.

15. Donald E. L. Johnson, ed., "Multi-Hospital System Survey," *Modern Healthcare,* April 1980, p. 57.

16. Sr. Mary Maurita Sengelaub, "Catholic Health Care Systems: A Sign of the Times," in Montague Brown and Barbara McCool, *Multihospital Systems: Strategies for Organization and Management* (Germantown, Md.: Aspen Systems Corp., 1980), p. 463.

17. Vince DiPaolo, "Adventists Hospital Groups Get the Urge to Merge," *Modern Healthcare,* October 1980, p. 56.

18. Robert Derzon, Lawrence S. Lewin, and J. Michael Watt, "Not-for-Profit Chains Share in Multihospital System Boom," *Hospitals,* May 16, 1981, p. 70.

19. Montague Brown, "Multihospital Systems: Trends, Issues, Prospects," prepared for HRET Invitational Conference on Multihospital Systems, Washington, D.C., March 18, 1980, p. 21.

20. Elworth Taylor, "Survey Shows Who Is Sharing Which Services," *Hospitals,* September 19, 1979.

7 Vertical integration

The second type of response of the hospital to intensifying market pressures is to integrate vertically (within the organization)—that is, through acquisitions and development of new forms of delivery of health care to capture and control more of the inputs which lead to inpatient hospitalization. As discussed earlier, vertical integration* in the hospital setting proceeded in two directions. As industrial firms integrated forward (toward the ultimate consumer of the firm's product), they either bought out the network of wholesale and, in some cases, retail distributors of their goods, or created their own distribution systems to bring their products to market. As they integrated backward (toward the supply of raw materials) they purchased either raw materials or primary producers of the goods needed to manufacture their products.

---

* The dimensions of integration are somewhat confusing. To integrate *horizontally* means to combine *across* business units, while to integrate *vertically* means to combine steps of production *within* the organization. The vertical dimension refers to the increased complexity of the product as it ascends through production to finished goods.

Vertical integration has a different meaning in the health care system. By far the most important "inputs" to the health care system are *people*—patients and the health professionals who serve them. Thus, vertical integration in a health enterprise involves linking together different levels of care and assembling the human resources needed to render that care. Only secondarily does integration in this setting mean procurement of goods or raw materials, which are an important, but not rate-limiting, factor in delivery of health care.

FORWARD INTEGRATION INTO AMBULATORY CARE

Since the hospital is the most highly organized form of production of health services, efforts by the hospital to reach those forms of care rendered to the patient prior to hospitalization can be considered forward integration—reaching out toward the patient. Most prehospital care is rendered in physicians' offices or in other primary practice settings (though in some cases, it can be rendered at home by nurses and allied health professionals). Forward integration from the hospital base generally means development of ambulatory care systems which relate, either formally or through collegial or medical ties, to the hospital.

In the industrial setting, the distribution system of a manufacturing firm comprises all the structures and intermediaries who guide the product to market. In the health care system it is the patient, not goods, which is mobile. Thus in health care the analog to distribution systems is that set of pathways and practitioners which result in bringing the patient to the hospital. This system is sometimes referred to as a "feeder system." The feeder system of a hospital includes all those settings in which the potential patient receives ambulatory services, or diagnosis, as well as the transportation systems and physician referral relationships which lead ultimately to hospitalization. Development of an effective feeder system is the principal marketing task of most hospitals.

For a number of years hospitals have employed a variety of strategies to bind the practice of ambulatory care more closely to the organization. To say that they were "pursuing a strategy of forward integration" makes some indefensible assumptions about the motives of those who planned the physicians' office buildings, ambulatory care centers, emergency rooms, and other facilities involved. In some cases these developments were intended to advance physician recruitment. In others they may have been planned to meet unmet community needs. In yet others they may have been part of an effort to increase hospital admissions from community physicians by providing them a convenient place to practice close to the hospital. The motives may well have varied. But the common element of the development of captive or hospital related ambulatory facilities has been to incorporate, physically or programmatically, more of the practice of medicine into the hospital setting. To the extent that any or all of these strategies have been pursued, they represented forward integration into ambulatory care.

The principal feeder system for most hospitals is the network of private offices and group practices where the hospital's medical staff renders ambulatory care. In most community hospitals, this network of private practices is beyond the corporate responsibility of the hospital and therefore the control of the hospital administrator. Rather, it is the exclusive province of the practicing physician. Efforts to involve the hospital more directly in the delivery of ambulatory care blur the boundaries of responsibility between the physician and hospital and, as will be seen later in the Chapter 8, create a fertile area of potential economic conflict.

Many hospitals analyze the origins of their patients. Yet relatively few hospital planners realize that the pattern of a hospital's primary service area is largely determined by where its voluntary medical staff practices, and in some cases where its members live. In the traditional, nonteaching hospital, this network of private physician offices was the hospital's only feeder system (Figure 7–1). The hospital's utilization was determined almost completely by the voluntary decisions of its medical staff to hospitalize patients at that hospital as opposed to competing facilities. In this type of hospital system the administrator is almost powerless to affect his facility's occupancy.

In contrast to this type of relationship, many of the nation's teaching hospitals and regional/national diagnostic centers, such as the Mayo and the Cleveland Clinics, have retained

FIGURE 7–1
Hospital feeder system, 1940

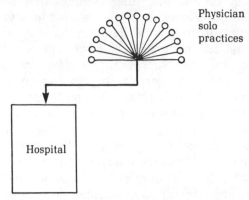

Physician solo practices

Hospital

physicians as salaried employees of the hospital. To push the analogy to the point of some unreality, this salaried arrangement comes the closest to the industrial analog of a salaried "sales force" under corporate control of the firm. By comparison, the traditional voluntary staff could be likened to a network of independent distributors. As discussed above, salaried, full-time medical staffs were vigorously attacked by private practicing physicians through their medical societies. Some tension along these lines remains to this day. Employment of a salaried medical staff is as far "forward" as an organization can move toward integrating physician practice into the organization. For reasons discussed below, however, it may be *too* far in tomorrow's health care market.

Large, organized outpatient departments were the traditional vehicle for delivering ambulatory care in the municipal hospitals and the large urban teaching hospitals. Many of these large clinics were staffed by residents or interns under varying degrees of supervision by the hospital's full-time attending physicians. As the conventional community hospital began to diversify, many of them developed outpatient clinic space in their facilities which was either rented or given gratis to members of their attending staff to practice ambulatory medicine onsite. In some cases the hospital provided clerical support to schedule appointments for these physicians.

Interestingly, a recent study of the relative roles of patients and physicians in initiating ambulatory visits suggested that physicians exert greater control over ambulatory use in the hospital outpatient department than in their own offices.

In the late 1940s and in the 1950s hospitals began to add emergency rooms—facilities where patients could be seen without appointment for urgent conditions. As physicians became less willing to see patients in their own homes, or became less accessible in their offices, emergency rooms became increasingly used as primary physicians of last resort for many conditions that were not acute emergencies. In inner-city areas which lost physicians as they deteriorated economically or changed racially, hospital emergency rooms took up the slack and became the primary physician for large populations of patients who had no family physicians. Initially, these facilities were staffed on a rotating basis by junior members of the hospital's medical staff, some of whom used the emergency room to build their practices. However, a new hospital-based specialty of emergency medicine has emerged whose physicians practice full-time in the emergency rooms. While many of these physicians serve as salaried members of the hospital staff, emergency rooms are increasingly staffed by groups, and in some cases corporations, under contract to the hospital.

Emergency rooms have become a major source of inpatient admissions to the hospital, accounting for from 15 to 30 percent of a typical hospital's inpatients. Because these admissions do not depend upon the physicians' prior decision to hospitalize a patient, so much as the patient's presentation to the hospital directly (either on his or her own volition or in an ambulance), emergency rooms provide a source of patients which is independent of the hospital's voluntary staff (though most ER admissions must be arranged through a member of the staff through an on-call list or some other means). The emergency room thus lessens the dependence of the hospital upon discretionary admitting decisions by members of its voluntary staff. (See Figure 7–2.)

The structure resulting from these developments (Figure 7–3) spreads the sources of potential inpatient admissions among several separate systems, some of which the hospital controls.

When it became clear that many physicians desired greater control over their clinical practices than was afforded

FIGURE 7–2
Type of visit in selected medical settings: Percent distribution of ambulatory physician visits (January–March 1977)

Type of visit	All	Physician's office	Hospital outpatient department	Hospital emergency room	Other medical setting*
Physician initiated (set by the physician in a previous visit)	36.4	36.3	50.7	6.2	39.6
Patient initiated (patient called for an appointment or walked in)	59.6	59.8	44.8	89.2	56.3
Unknown	4.0	3.9	4.6	4.6	4.1
Total	100.0	100.0	100.0	100.0	100.0

* Includes military clinics, school clinics, and neighborhood health clinics or centers.
Source: U.S. Department of Health and Human Services, Public Health Service, Office of Health Research, Statistics and Technology, National Center for Health Services Research, 1977.

by hospital outpatient departments, hospitals began to construct physicians' office buildings adjacent to their facilities to house private practices. In other cases the hospital encouraged its physicians to construct such facilities themselves or to convert nearby residences to offices. In most instances where the hospital owns the facility, it leases space to the

FIGURE 7–3
Hospital feeder system, 1960

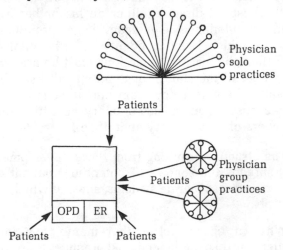

physicians who use the building. Sometimes these lease costs are temporarily subsidized by the hospital (e.g., for physicians starting up their practices). The physical proximity of the office building encourages physicians who may maintain other offices near their homes or with colleagues to use the hospital.

Control over leases affords the hospital administrator some measure of control over aspects of clinical practice. For example, lease provisions may prevent physicians from competing with certain of the hospital's clinical services (e.g., laboratory and radiology). Administrators may also decline to renew leases for physicians who fail to hospitalize a significant percentage of the patients at the facility.

This nominal power may disappear, however, if a new trend in physician's office building management becomes more widespread. Many hospitals which own their own office buildings have begun converting them to condominiums and selling space to physician tenants. This not only provides the hospital with ready, unencumbered cash but also relieves it of the management responsibilities and associated maintenance costs of operating the building. Concurrently, the purchase of the space provides the physician considerable tax advantages, particularly if he or she is incorporated.

By the late 1960s, many hospitals began constructing satellite office buildings and ambulatory care facilities remote from the original hospital site. The purpose of this branching is to provide the hospital a physician presence in developing areas. The development of satellites reflected a growing awareness that the location of the primary physician's office was becoming increasingly important to the patient, and that concentrating ambulatory services around the hospital site might limit access of patients who move into other parts of the community. This strategy was particularly popular for inner city hospitals whose physicians began to be concerned about the viability of their practices in the face of racial or socioeconomic change.

In some cases, satellite office buildings and ambulatory facilities gave way to satellite *hospitals*. The concept of a satellite hospital is troublesome, since its use may cut into that of the core hospital, cannibalizing the core hospital's market. Avoiding the cannibalization of existing markets by new branches is a perennial problem in commercial retailing. Medical staff who live in developing areas may reduce their use of the core facility for routine care if closer facilities are available. Even owning the satellite hospital may not be enough to prevent its natural evolution into a competitor, particularly if the market for physicians in the outlying area is sufficiently competitive.

As discussed in the chapter on health maintenance, some larger hospitals have established health maintenance organizations. The HMO will usually contract with the hospital to serve the HMO's patients on an inpatient basis. However, the establishment of an HMO by a hospital inevitably involves an economic conflict of interest. Owing to the HMO's imperative to minimize hospitalization, the development of a captive HMO may not be an intelligent outreach strategy. However, as HMO enrollment grows in particular communities, hospitals with excess capacity may look to HMOs as a source of patients, providing that they can render cost-effective inpatient care at a price both the HMO and the hospital can afford. Though HMOs will not provide the quantum of inpatient volume that a conventional ambulatory care facility or group practice will (per given volume of outpatient visits), it may make sense to include HMOs as a component of a hospital's feeder system in tightening markets.

For the teaching or referral hospital, the community-based practices of primary physicians in the area or region also constitute a portion of the feeder system. Referrals from community-based practitioners are an important source of patients for the tertiary level teaching hospital. Since the complexity of care in teaching centers is typically higher than in a community hospital, developing clinical cooperation with community institutions is also forward integration. Medical staffs of community-based facilities rightfully expect that patients sent to tertiary hospitals for diagnosis or therapy to be returned to them for continuing care. However, they are also beginning to demand referral of less complex cases inappropriate to the high cost teaching hospital setting in return. They may also demand attending or consulting privileges at the teaching facility as well as academic appointments. To the extent that referrals into the tertiary center take place, the community hospitals and their medical staffs become part of the feeder systems of the tertiary hospital.

The consequence of all of these developments is that feeder systems for hospitals have diversified to the point when hospitals have multiple sources of inpatients (Figure 7–4). The fact that the hospital does not control all of them is not as important as the diversity itself. To the extent that hospitals depend on a variety of sources of patients, they spread their risks and dilute the power of any one group of physician or organized providers to determine their operating positions. Thus, it is in a hospital's interests to diversify the sources of potential inpatients.

The degree of control the hospital should exert over the organizations which feed the hospital may present a reimbursement dilemma for the hospital manager. For example, to the degree that captive ambulatory facilities are part of the hospital's cost base for accounting and reimbursement purposes, they can reduce the level of reimbursement for

FIGURE 7–4
Hospital feeder system, 1980

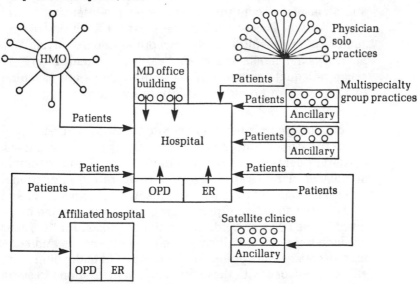

the core inpatient facility. More will be said about this problem below in the discussion of corporate restructuring.

But a far more serious problem relates to the incursion of the hospital into the economic turf of the practicing physician. Hospital control over ambulatory services may pose an economic threat to the private practices of its own medical staff, creating a managerial and political dilemma of major proportions for the hospital. In the chapter on ambulatory care, it was established that these ambulatory practices will be increasingly stressed economically as the supply of physicians increases. The issue of how far forward the hospital should integrate into ambulatory care will be discussed in Chapter 8. The resolution of this conflict of economic interests between the physician and the hospital may be one of the most difficult managerial dilemmas facing hospital managers, trustees, and physicians in the future market for health care.

BACKWARD INTEGRATION

In the industrial setting, backward integration involves all those activities the firm engages in to secure an adequate supply of the raw materials needed for manufacture. In the health care setting, the product is a human service. Hospitals and other health care providers are people-intensive operations. As will be seen later, the most critically scarce resources of the hospital are its own professionals: physicians, nurses, technicians, and other health personnel. Efforts to secure adequate supplies of these individuals are essential to a health care provider's ability to function.

For many years, hospitals operated their own nursing programs to assure themselves a steady supply of trained nurses. Hospital operated nursing programs are a classic example of backward integration. However, operating educational programs of any kind in a hospital setting is expensive, and many of the so-called diploma programs have become casualties of the drive to contain health care costs. As the focus of nurse training shifts increasingly to universities and community colleges, hospitals will be compelled to develop more effective liaisons with these educational institutions to serve as training sites. Providing training opportunities for nurses gives the hospital a recruitment advantage over nonaffiliated institutions.

At the same time, many hospitals have operated residency training programs for physicians beyond the MD level to train in particular medical specialties. By establishing these programs, hospitals can secure a captive market of potential recruits to the medical staff. In recent years the federal government became increasingly interested in encouraging the growth of residency programs in so-called primary care specialties, such as pediatrics, family practice, obstetrics, and gynecology. The physicians trained in these specialties have a special attraction for the hospital administrator, since they must depend heavily on consultation from specialty colleagues on the hospital's medical staff for management of complex medical problems. Patients requiring surgery or complex diagnostic procedures will be referred from the primary practitioner to hospital specialists, augmenting the hospital's activity levels (whether ambulatory or inpatient). Attracting primary care specialists to the hospital's staff through residency training not only enables the hospital to develop new markets of primary care patients through the new physician practices, but assures a flow of patients to subspecialists if these patients become acutely ill.

Unfortunately, expansion of these primary care residency programs may be curtailed by tightening federal resources for health care. In this case hospitals will consider establishing relationships with established medical school based residency programs. These relationships provide that the hospital will serve as a training site for residents rotating from the medical school's principal teaching hospital. These rotations are important educational experiences for the resident, since community-based hospitals offer a different type of milieu and practice setting than most teaching hospitals and help prepare the specialist for actual medical practice. The rotations also provide the hospital an opportunity to recruit the residents by exposing them to collegial ties and practice opportunities in the hospital's neighborhood or region.

These educational affiliations have an important spinoff for the community hospital's administration and medical staff. Participation in university-based teaching programs may qualify the community hospital's physicians for university academic appointments (such as clinical professorships). The appointments may be important to community physicians, providing them referral ties and points of entry to the teaching hospital as well as prestige in the community. The ability of administrators to offer such opportunities through affiliation with medical schools may help in medical staff recruitment or in stabilizing existing members of the medical staff.

Some hospitals and multihospital systems have considered integrating backward into medical supplies and other goods needed to operate the hospital. In doing so, however, these organizations may be entering well established, highly organized, and competitive markets dominated by large firms. Most hospital supply companies are high volume, low margin operations which require extensive distribution systems and marketing expertise as well as research and development activities to make them successful. Even large hospital management firms will think twice before entering these markets. The risks of integrating backward into the medical supply business seem far to outweigh the possible benefits. Such endeavors as joint purchasing make far more sense than developing new lines of business in the medical supply area.

DEVELOPMENT OF TRANSPORTATION SYSTEMS

The most difficult logistical problem for hospitals is to accommodate the mobility of the patient by escaping the geographical constraint of a single, core physical plant. There are two ways to do this. The first, discussed earlier, is to develop satellite ambulatory facilities which serve the desired market area. Outlets for the hospital's or medical staff's services which are closer to the desired patient population than the core hospital help solve the problem of access by coming to the patient.

The other strategy, which is less expensive, is to develop captive transportation systems to bring the patient to the hospital. Many hospitals have recognized the importance of accessibility of their facility by constructing parking structures adjacent to the hospital for convenience to the patient and the medical staff. But a bolder step is to develop vehicles and systems to convey patients to the hospital directly.

Some larger organizations have developed imaginative transportation systems. The University of Iowa Hospitals and Clinics have developed such a system. The University Hospitals are an 1,100-bed facility located in Iowa City, a town of approximately 60,000 people. In order to survive, the hospital cannot rely on utilization by the local community and must reach out to the entire state. To accomplish this objective, they developed a fleet of Checker limousines which can be dispatched from Iowa City to any location in the state to bring patients to the hospital. This service has made it much more convenient for Iowa's physicians to rely on the tertiary level medical services at the University of Iowa, which is *the* tertiary medical center for the state.

Another organization which has made a major investment in transportation systems is the Samaritan Health Service of Phoenix, one of the nation's most successful secular non-profit multihospital systems. Samaritan operates a fixed-wing air ambulance which brings patients in from the isolated regions of northern Arizona and New Mexico. These regions contain major recreational areas as well as mining and energy development projects which produce a significant amount of medical trauma. In cooperation with a smaller freestanding hospital in the area, Samaritan also has developed a helicopter transportation service to provide direct access to remote accident sites which cannot be reached by the fixed-wing service. The helicopter service has been sufficiently successful that Samaritan is contemplating acquiring a second aircraft to meet additional demand. Both the fixed-wing and helicopter systems are equipped with life-support equipment and carry a critical care nurse who is linked to the core Good Samaritan Hospital by radiotelemetry for medical consultation.

In addition to its air ambulances, Samaritan has developed a fleet of mobile intensive care vans, which are used to transport patients requiring sophisticated diagnostic procedures from the service's community-based facilities to Good Samaritan Hospital. Patients are transported to Good Samaritan for the procedure and are returned quickly to the hospital of origin with the diagnostic results for their physician to review. This system has been helpful in increasing utilization of the Good Samaritan CAT scanner and other high technology diagnostic equipment. Samaritan recently moved to acquire a local ambulance company to expand service to its system on a 24-hour basis. The company will continue to service other hospitals according to the protocols of the Phoenix emergency services system, but will be able as well to convey patients referred from network hospitals to Good Samaritan.

Hospitals contemplating development of captive transportation systems face some political and regulatory problems from ambulance and taxi companies as well as from competing hospitals. Ambulance companies often have considerable leeway in where they take the critically ill patient. If captive systems are perceived to be competitors, established independent ambulance companies may discontinue serving the core hospital's emergency room to the extent that local Emergency Medical Service (EMS) protocols permit. For this reason Samaritan has explicitly linked its mobile intensive care vans to network hospitals and will not pick patients up at accident sites or their homes. To the extent that hospitals get into the ambulance business directly they expose themselves to common-carrier regulation and may require licensure by city agencies. Nevertheless, diversification into transportation services is an imaginative approach to escaping the geographical constraints of a core physical plant which helps make the hospital's services accessible to patients and physicians.

A VERTICALLY INTEGRATED HOSPITAL SYSTEM

One of the most sophisticated organizational structures developed by a hospital, which encompasses both horizontal and vertical integration, may be found at Rush Presbyterian-St Lukes Hospital and Medical Center in Chicago. Over a decade ago, under the leadership of Dr. James Campbell, a forceful, articulate health care innovator, Rush embarked upon an organizational strategy which has given rise to a structure not dissimilar to a modern multidivisional corporation. The core hospital contains approximately 873 beds, located in an inner-city area on the west side of Chicago adjacent to the University of Illinois Medical Center and the Cook County Hospital. The owned portion of the Rush system also includes a 138-bed inpatient hospital on the lake-front and a 176-bed geriatric facility on the Rush campus, for a total of 1,187 beds.

The Medical Center budget, including its educational and research programs, was approximately $220 million for the 1980–81 fiscal year. If one includes the 11 hospitals with which Rush is affiliated or associated, the total beds in the Rush system amount to 5,116. Only two nonprofit systems in the country exceed it in bed size (Kaiser and Sisters of Mercy).

The strategy which guided the diversification of the system was based on the principle that the system should serve comprehensively the health care needs of approximately 1.5 million persons. That is, the system should generate the health care personnel and coordinate the health care services at all levels—ambulatory and inpatient—for the people in this population. The system was to be constructed nongeo-graphically, in the sense that the population to be served would not be confined to a particular set of boundaries but be spread throughout a region (the Chicago metropolitan area and northern Illinois).

To accomplish the health personnel component, it was necessary to integrate backwards into the supply of health manpower. In 1969 Dr. Campbell reactivated the long dor-mant Rush Medical College (formerly linked to the Universiy of Chicago). Using state and federal aid to health education as building blocks, he built the program into a university for the health sciences with three colleges (medicine, nursing and allied health). The medical college had an enrollment of 479 students in 1979, the majority of whom are drawn from Illinois. In addition, 341 MD's are engaged in medical education at the post-MD (residency) level. These residency programs were originally freestanding under hospital spon-sorship and were brought under the auspices of the medical college. Of the residents trained in the system, approximately 40 percent are retained within the system upon completion of their training. Residents are exposed to practice opportunities in affiliated institutions and are encouraged (in a low-key way) to practice in the region.

The students in the Rush programs in the nursing and allied health professions also represent a substantial captive market of potential recruits into the Rush system. Recent retention rates within Rush for nursing graduates approach 60 percent, critically important in the increasingly tight nursing market. Of the nurses retained, approximately two thirds work at the core Presbyterian St. Lukes Hospital.

In addition to generating health personnel for its system and the patients it serves, the Rush academic programs, supported by clinical research activities, helps Rush retain its clinical faculty and medical staff and recruit high quality residents into its specialty training programs. The ability to grant academic appointments in the college of medicine has facilitated the development of affiliations with community based institutions. These institutions serve as sites for residency training and medical student clerkships, broadening the clinical experience beyond the tertiary hospital to primary and secondary care in the community setting.

The second major component of the Rush corporate plan involved development of a diversified ambulatory care distribution system to feed the core metropolitan area. During the late 1960s, under separate incorporation, Rush launched two health care programs—the Mile Square Health Center and the Anchor Organization for Health Maintenance. The former organization is a network of inner city ambulatory care facilities affiliated with Rush Medical College. It delivers approximately 140,000 outpatient visits annually. The Anchor HMO is a staff model HMO which had achieved an enrollment of 38,000 persons in 1980. Medical staff in both organizations have faculty appointments in the Rush Medical College.

In addition to these two programs, Rush constructed a physicians' office building with capacity for 200 practicing physicians adjacent to the core hospital. This building houses many of the medical practices of the Rush medical staff as well as facilities for outpatient ancillary services (radiology and clinical laboratories) and outpatient surgery, and a branch of the Anchor HMO. The facility was almost immediately filled, and plans are being made to double the physicians' office capacity by adding a second building.

Having put this diversified structure in place Dr. Campbell closed the hospital's outpatient department, which he considered to be an obsolete and excessively costly method of rendering care. The core hospital relies on referrals from the various feeder mechanisms and from physicians in affiliated and other community hospitals, and on a small emergency room (Cook County's vast emergency facilities are 100 yards away) to keep the hospital full. Both the Anchor and Miles Square physicians are encouraged to refer cases requiring routine, as opposed to tertiary hospitalization, to network hospitals to hold down the cost of care.

In addition to diversification into ambulatory care, Rush opened the luxurious 176-bed, Bowman Geriatric Hospital and chronic care facility on the Rush campus in 1976. Though it was intended to care for older individuals who are undergoing lengthy recuperation from illness, it can also serve as a residential or skilled nursing facility. Because of the facility's high costs, reflecting both intensity of the services provided and the amenities, it must rely on a private pay population. This facility enables Rush to make more effective use of its acute care beds by shifting patients into the Bowman facility.

The third major component of the strategy was the development of a network of affiliations with community-based facilities in the region. Most of these facilities are concentrated in the western suburbs of Chicago, though there are several large inner-city affiliates. The primary axis of the affiliations is medical education. Through the relationship, medical staffs of affiliated institutions receive faculty appointments at Rush Medical College and are encouraged to use the expensive tertiary level medical services available at Rush (open heart surgery, kidney transplant, perinatal care, etc.) by referring patients requiring subspecialty care or consultation to the core hospital.

According to Dr. Campbell, the watchword of these relationships is "voluntarism." Dr. Campbell has not demanded
a role in program planning at the affiliated institutions, and
has no role in budgetary matters or executive or medical
staffing decisions at these institutions, though he does exercise considerable informal influence over some key decisions. Several of the wealthier affiliates have developed their
own tertiary level programs and services and do not avail
themselves of the core hospital's services to a great extent.
Where the waiting lists for elective surgery at Rush have
grown too lengthy, development of satellite programs in network facilities has been encouraged. The core hospital has
operated at or near its capacity for some time, and does
not have the capacity to absorb all or even the majority of
the referrals generated from the 4,000-bed network of affiliates.

The strength of the network does not derive from the corporate relationships and agreements between administrators
of the constituent hospitals in the Rush system. Rather, to
the extent that it functions as a system, it does so by virtue
of preexisting collegial ties between the medical staffs of
affiliated institutions, many of whom are loyal alumni of
the Presbyterian-St. Lukes residency programs which pre-
dated the establishment of the Rush Medical College. It is
through these ties that referrals flow to the Center.

Because it is a nonprofit corporation and one which must
protect vulnerable medical education and research programs
through endowments and grant support, it is unlikely that
the Rush system will be able to generate the capital to aug-
ment the *owned* portion. The 110-bed Sheridan Road Pavil-
lion on the lakefront was donated to Rush and has been
something of a financial drain on the system. However, Dr.
Campbell holds out the possibility that some affiliated institutions may become sufficiently comfortable with the relationship that they may elect to merge with the core hospital.

During the late 1970s, Rush developed a separately incorporated for-profit managment company called BioServices,
Inc. The original intention of this firm was to involve itself
in contract management of health facilities in the region with
the potential of doubling the number of beds, both acute

and long-term care, linked to Rush. After some initial problems in the long-term care field, the firm retargeted itself to shared management systems and services. But through BioServices, Rush retains the capability of diversifying into contract management and extending its reach into other states.

The Rush network has been able to compete very effectively in an intensely competitive tertiary marketplace in the Chicago area, which is a regional referral center for the Midwest. Through its board and administrators, Rush has had a major influence on the evolution of health care policy at the local and state levels. At one point during the 1970s, the chief of the state health department and the chief health planner for Illinois were both senior administrators in the Rush system. These political ties also played an important role in developing the system itself, as Dr. Campbell developed an excellent working relationship with Chicago's late Mayor Richard Daley and his administration.

The structure resulting from this ambitious corporate strategy has effectively achieved Dr. Campbell's initial objectives. It has virtually reached the population level of 1.5 million he intended to serve and has assured a solvent, successful core hospital. If funds for medical education are reduced, the clinical operations of the Rush system will be sufficiently strong to absorb an increasing share of the burden of financing health education, though Dr. Campbell remains comfortable with this type of cross subsidization.

The System is not without problems—relationships with neighboring and affiliated institutions have not always gone smoothly. Dr. Campbell has not had a comfortable relationship with his immediate public hospital neighbors, the University of Illinois and Cook County Hospital. Despite the fact that County's vast ambulatory services have relieved community-service pressure from the core Rush Presbyterian-St. Lukes Hospital, Dr. Campbell has advocated the closure of County Hospital for many years on the ground that it perpetuated a two-class system of health care.

Even though some of its operations, such as the Bowman Geriatric Center, have lost money or had unanticipated lengthy start-up phases, the overall system is healthy. The Rush system is a model of cooperative and managed multi-institutional relationships which can provide a vehicle for linking health resources together to assure the survival of constituent elements. Rush is better protected than its competitors from major shifts in the reimbursement system or in demand for patient care services. Since it does not own all the elements of the system, but works with them through cooperative programs, it has successfully spread its risks over a very large health care network.

STRUCTURAL ALTERNATIVES FOR THE FREESTANDING HOSPITAL

Since it has proven politically impossible to control health costs by regulating physician practice, government efforts to constrain health care spending have inevitably been directed at the least mobile target, the hospital. As a result, community hospital administrators and trustees encounter a daunting maze of regulatory constraints on their activities. Some of these constraints, such as the reimbursement rules of Medicare and Medicaid, have seriously eroded hospitals' capital base and discouraged efforts to diversify and develop new sources of revenue and methods of delivering health care.

Nevertheless, some innovative hospital administrators have found methods of escaping some of these constraints by developing new corporate structures which segregate the regulated lines of health care business from other potential growth activities. The legal and accounting issues surrounding corporate structure are bewilderingly complex and are well beyond the purview of this book. However, it is important to realize that multihospital strategies are not the only alternative for hospitals desiring to remain competitive and financially viable in a tightening market.

The objective of corporate restructuring is to provide a corporate framework which permits administrators and boards of trustees to insulate revenues from new health care ventures, philanthropy, and other revenue-generating activity from regulation directed at core health care delivery functions. If new structures are not created to segregate such income, it can either be declared taxable or offset against the hospital's patient care reimbursement by Medicaid and Medicare. Since the principal financial problem of hospitals in a competitive environment may be access to capital and preservation of the hospital's capital base, sheltering income from new ventures becomes a near paramount concern.

There are enumerable permutations of possible new structures, but the common element of these structures seems to be submerging the hospital in a multicorporation superstructure, where the controlling organization is not a health care enterprise (e.g., a foundation or other corporate organization). Thus, the hospital becomes a *subsidiary* of an enterprise which has no direct responsibility for delivering health care. The controlling organization may hold title to hospital fixed assets, or the hospital's endowment, and control the dispersement of its proceeds or related philanthropy.

By creating a nonhealth care delivery enterprise to control the hospital, lines of business which operate in price-sensitive markets (e.g., markets where insurance coverage is either thin or nonexistent) can be spun off from the hospital as separate corporations but kept under common supervision. Medicare and Medicaid reimbursement principles conspire to drive up the cost of ambulatory care, for example, by requiring unreasonable overhead allocations to such activities. By spinning off these activities, particularly those in satellites, rates for ambulatory care can be held down and, correspondingly, reimbursement for inpatient services in the core facility can be preserved or even increased. The superstructure also permits creation of for-profit subsidiaries whose revenues, while taxable, may not offset reimbursement for health services delivered by the hospital.

A recent example of corporate restructuring based upon a single freestanding hospital was the reorganization of Lutheran General Hospital in Park Ridge, Illinois. Under the leadership of George Caldwell this 800-bed facility restructured itself and placed the hospital under one of two not-for-profit holding companies (see Figure 7–5). The underlying logic of the restructuring was to create two holding companies, the Lutheran Institute of Human Ecology to hold the regulated health enterprises subject to health planning and

FIGURE 7-5
Corporate organization chart

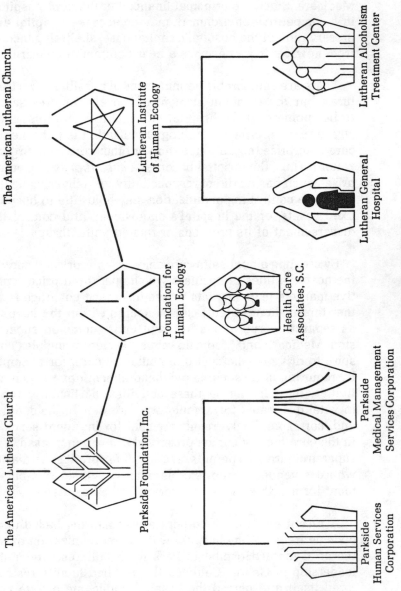

The American Lutheran Church

The American Lutheran Church

Parkside Foundation, Inc.

Foundation for Human Ecology

Lutheran Institute of Human Ecology

Parkside Human Services Corporation

Parkside Medical Management Services Corporation

Health Care Associates, S.C.

Lutheran General Hospital

Lutheran Alcoholism Treatment Center

Source: Reprinted by permission, Lutheran General Hospital, Park Ridge, Illinois.

Medicare/Medicaid oversight, and The Parkside Foundation to hold the nonregulated revenue-generating growth businesses which Caldwell has identified as the future "endowment" of the hospital.

The Parkside Foundation will foster the development of a number of health related businesses which are targeted to areas of identified market potential. The Parkside Human Services Corporation will manage the hospital's freestanding ambulatory care facility, which was spun off from the hospital proper; its pastoral counselling and outpatient psychiatric services; and the hospital's unique network of outreach facilities, which Caldwell terms "ecology centers." Physicians' services in all these enterprises are billed through an independent professional corporation.

The ecology center will be based on the "wellness" concept, which involves treating patient problems more broadly than through medical intervention. Linked to clergy in specific target communities, these centers will incorporate primary physicians, pastoral counsellors, and other professionals to encourage spiritual and psychological as well as physical health. The centers will serve as auxiliaries to the primary practice sites of physicians who trained in Lutheran General's residency programs, and who will practice in the community, though remaining linked to Lutheran General for tertiary care referrals and continuing medical education.

The second principal "growth" business sheltered by the Parkside Foundation is a diversified consulting enterprise, Parkside Medical Services Corporation, headed by a former vice chairman of the Arthur Andersen accounting firm. Though the firm will conduct traditional hospital consulting activities, its principal lines of business will be the development of owned and managed alcohol treatment centers, both freestanding and hospital-based, and health benefits management services targeted to corporations. The goal of the latter line of business will be to offer a comprehensive set of management services aimed at reducing a corporation's health care outlays. These two lines of business are intended to build from the large regional base of the Chicago area to national markets. Through an intermediate Foundation for Human Ecology, proceeds of these nonhospital activities may be channelled back to Lutheran General Hospital as needed to help preserve its role as a tertiary care teaching hospital in an increasingly hostile reimbursement and funding climate.

Caldwell's strategy may provide Lutheran General the capital resources to weather significant changes in the reimbursement system, or permit it to grow or diversify if capital markets for hospitals tighten. In the process, Caldwell has developed a corporate structure which, while remaining health care related, has enabled him to diversify into nonmedical services in areas of major market opportunity. If these nonmedical lines of business prove sufficiently successful, his structure provides him the flexibility to take them public and enter the equity markets to which not-for-profit organizations currently do not have access. As Caldwell has argued, survival in a tightening market is not enough. For those with entrepreneurial energy, and the support of their board and medical staff, innovation may lead to success and to control of new health-related markets for health services.

While different in their structure and motivation, the Rush and Lutheran General corporate strategies have some common elements. Growing outward from a core hospital, they transform the hospital into a division of a diversified health care enterprise. They permit penetration of multiple markets and control over wide geographical areas. The multiple structures permit a wide variety of subsidy arrangements and maximize opportunities to compete in price-sensitive markets by segregating those activities corporately from cost-reimbursed services. They also help maximize physician income by breaking physician reimbursement out of the hospital cost matrix, permitting physicians to be reimbursed at full charges through private practice corporations.

These strategies represent the wave of the future for hospital organization. They demonstrate only two of a myriad of possible creative approaches to integration and diversification and represent imaginative attempts to solve legal and regulatory problems facing hospitals. To be sure, there are major uncertainties about these new organizations, including their credit worthiness and the response of reimbursing and taxing bodies to them. While these corporate strategies are legally and managerially complex, they have a degree of flexibility which permits the organization to adapt and to protect its most vulnerable element, the hospital, from abrupt or damaging shifts in the competitive or financial environment. Those organizations which have undergone such transformations resemble structurally the corporations which reached Chandler's fourth stage of evolution of business organization and seem to be exceptionally well equipped to compete effectively in the tightening health care market.

8

Physician and the hospital

The preceding chapter makes clear that one of the principal strategies of hospitals facing market pressures from competing hospitals is to integrate forward into ambulatory care—that is, to try to control more prehospital medical care to assure that patients requiring hospital care come to their facility.

By integrating forward into ambulatory care, however, hospitals may move into direct competition with their own medical staff's practices which, as we discussed in the chapter on ambulatory care, are under increasing competitive pressure. These two simultaneous developments could aggravate an inherent conflict of interest between the hospital and its medical staff. Since hospitals are a delicate balance of institutional and medical interests, aggravation of this conflict could damage both the institution and the physicians who rely upon it. This chapter will discuss the nature of the potential economic conflict and suggest some remedies for it.

PHYSICIAN VERSUS ADMINISTRATIVE PERSPECTIVES
ON THE ROLE OF THE HOSPITAL

Hospitals do not admit patients into their facilities; its physicians do. Physicians incorporate the hospital and its resources into the management of their patients. Physicians (as well as hospital boards of trustees) are held legally responsible for the quality of medical care and, under accreditation requirements, for assuring the quality of care rendered by their colleagues. Medical staffs function as largely self-governing entities within the supportive framework of the hospital. Physicians judge the hospital by the extent to which it supports or impedes their medical practice as well as by their patients' perception of the facility. What infuriates physicians about hospitals and their administrators more than anything else is the encroachment of bureaucratic constraints and administrative inadequacies on their ability to deliver quality care to their patients. These bureaucratic constraints are frequently the product of reimbursement and regulatory systems which require accountability for resource consumption, and of the fact that hospital resources are limited. They are sometimes worsened by hospital administrators who have lost sight of the fact that the physician is the true market for the hospital's services.

Physicians determine how and how much hospitals are used. In those hospitals which have voluntary (e.g., nonsalaried) staffs, the physician alone decides how much he or she wishes to use the hospital. Many physicians are members of more than one hospital medical staff. Because physician fees (under fee-for-service) and hospital costs are reimbursed separately for most physician care, physician fees flow directly to the physician regardless of where he or she hospitalizes patients. Physicians who are dissatisfied with the support they are receiving at one hospital may elect to take their business (*and* the hospital revenues they generate) to a competing facility. The amount of use of various facilities is dependent on where the physician has privileges and on bed and operating room availability at the various hospitals, as well as how supportive the physician feels the hospital is of his or her practice.

As the hospital administrator confronts the changing health care environment, that person labors under some

unique managerial constraints. While the hospital administrator has unambiguous responsibility for the core hotel management functions of the hospital, such as billing and
collection, admitting, housekeeping, materiel management,
and the laundry, the administrator has almost no ability directly to control the utilization of the hospital's services.
The administrator can *influence* that utilization indirectly
by running a more efficient operation than competitors, by
responding, within fiscal and legal limits, to the needs of
the medical staff and by fostering a climate of cooperation.
But an administrator cannot compel physicians to bring patients to the hospital. Having no control over the incomes
of admitters in the vast majority of cases, the administrator
cannot discourage physicians from withdrawing their business and taking it to competitors. A hospital administrator's
power lies in the ability to command the respect and support
of the medical staff. The necessity of accomplishing this difficult political task while simultaneously guarding the hospital's fiscal condition is what makes the job almost impossible.

As hospital administrators and physicians attempt to develop strategies to cope with their respective competitive
environments, there are likely to be several areas where
their interests diverge, creating the potential for conflict.
These areas will be discussed below and, as a conclusion,
some thoughts on how to resolve the conflicts will be offered.

PHYSICIAN COMPENSATION

As a general principle, the closer a hospital administrator
comes to "controlling" what a physician earns, the more
heat is likely to be generated by the relationship. As discussed earlier, fee-for-service billing permits the physician
maximum discretion over the conduct of his or her practice
and offers minimum capacity for administrative intrusion
in physician activities. However, a significant minority of
physicians in the United States (approximately 28 percent[1])
are not compensated through fee-for-service but are salaried
employees of the hospital. Moreover, many physicians are
contractors to the hospital, delivering services under a wide
variety of compensation schemes. These physicians are frequently referred to as "hospital-based physicians," though
many so-called hospital-based physicians retain the preroga-
tive to bill patients directly for their care.

Most hospital-based specialists require a hospitalized patient population to generate their incomes. Generically, hospital-based physicians can be distinguished from other physicians in that they do not *admit* patients to the hospital. They must rely on practitioners who are capable of bringing their patients into the hospital, who generically are called "admitting physicians." The admitting physicians of a hospital are the portion of its medical staff which functions as its "sales force." Some admitting physicians such as cardiologists, neurologists, and pulmonary medicine specialists may be retained by the hospital under contract to interpret the results of diagnostic tests such as EEGs and EKGs, but the relationship does not extend to the physician's activities as an admitter. Except in teaching hospitals and public/general hospitals, admitting physicians are rarely contractual employees of the hospital, and overwhelmingly, bill on a fee-for-service basis.

The methods of compensation of hospital-based specialists are a subject of general controversy for several reasons. These revenues are not an insignificant fraction (5 to 9 percent) of all hospital costs.[2] Some economists have called hospital-based physicians "franchised monopolists" since their relationship to the hospital guarantees them revenues from whatever ancillary activity the hospital generates. Hospital-based physician incomes are also much higher than those of office-based medical specialists, though there are major income disparities depending on the nature of the compensation arrangement. In his review article on this subject, Bruce Steinwald found that

> hospital-based practice is considerably more lucrative than office-based, on the average. Estimated mean net income per hour of medical activity in 1976–77 ranged from 15 percent higher for anaesthesiologists to 53 percent higher for radiologists. On a per hour basis, fee-for-service is the most lucrative form of HBP compensation, followed closely by percentage of department revenue and not so closely by salaried compensation.[3]

According to Steinwald, since the enactment of Medicare, compensation arrangements have moved away from revenue sharing with hospital departments (so-called percentage arrangements) to separate, fee-for-service billing. Congressional actions may eventually prohibit the percentage arrangement where physicians share in a percentage or gross or net departmental revenues. These arrangements are felt to have encouraged excessive use of ancillary services, and contributed disproportionately to increasing health care costs. As Steinwald has pointed out, however, research findings on the impact of various compensation mechanisms on physician productivity are virtually nonexistent, complicating dialogue about how to reform the reimbursement system.[4]

From a managerial point of view, arrangements with hospital based physicians can be arrayed along a continuum of control and managerial oversight, as in Figure 8–1. Salary arrangements entangle the administrator in difficult negotiations over appropriate salary levels for the service chief and his colleagues, where salary increases must be traded off against other items in the budget. However, salary discussions do permit surfacing of productivity and cost control issues, providing an administrator some opportunity for bargaining.

Salaried arrangements also encourage greater physician involvement in the administrative activities of the hospital, such as committee work. Because the practice takes place within the confines of the hospital, salaried physicians may have a greater commitment to broader institutional agendas which transcend their particular areas of practice.[5]

Clearly, however, salaried physicians inevitably confront the fact that they are *employees* of the hospital and in an employee-employer relationship with its administrator. Medical practitioners are generically hostile to subordination of their practices to nonphysicians. For this reason physicians prefer relationships which protect the independence of private medical practice, such as those in which the physician has the status of an independent contractor.

FIGURE 8–1
Continuum of physician compensation arrangements

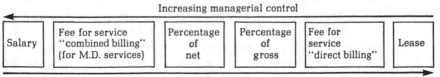

		Increasing managerial control			
Salary	Fee for service "combined billing" (for M.D. services)	Percentage of net	Percentage of gross	Fee for service "direct billing"	Lease

Increasing physician control

While percentage arrangements generally contain incentives to run active departments, they are, as mentioned above, amenable to abuse. Under the "percentage" concept the hospital guarantees the hospital-based physician either a fixed percentage of gross billings of the department or a fixed percentage of gross billings, net of expenses. The latter arrangement is thought to provide a greater physician incentive to control nonphysician costs (labor and materials), implicating the physician more directly in the hospital administrator's battle to control costs.[6] However, the percentage of net arrangement opens up a fertile ground for continuing conflict over such matters as the allocation of expenses to the department. Sometimes these percentages arrangements are negotiated with a guaranteed minimum income, which protects the physician but exposes the administrator if volume drops below a certain level. Guaranteed minimums rob the hospital administrator of the ability to control outlays if productivity falls off (that is, until the contract is subject to renegotiation).

Under percentage arrangements, generally, technicians and clerical staff remain employees of the hospital, and capital and personnel needs are negotiated with hospital administration. Under a lease arrangement the hospital leases space and equipment to a medical practitioner who in turn hires physicians and support staff independent of the hospital. The physician, directly or through a corporation, is responsible both for billing and collection for services and completely controls the budget, personnel policies, and productivity of his or her department. The cost of space and specific support services are clearly specified in the typical lease. These are the only financial transactions between physician and hospital. Under such arrangements the hospital administrator surrenders control almost completely to the physician.[7]

Under fee-for-service arrangements, the hospital may bill for the physician's professional fee along with hospital charges for particular ancillary procedures (so-called combined billing) or may bill solely for the hospital portion and permit the physician to bill the patient directly for physician services. The latter arrangement keeps physician income largely confidential from the hospital administrator. It also disentangles the physician from hospital data systems and the hospital's accounts receivable. This arrangement most closely approximates the billing status of the admitting physicians on the medical staff and conforms to the historic split between Blue Cross-Blue Shield and Medicare Part A/Part B services. The former arrangement, combined billing, where the hospital bills for the physicians as part of a combined MD-hospital charge, makes the total revenue generated by the hospital's ancillary departments a subject of managerial oversight and yields some greater measure of administrative control.

As discussed in the chapter on vertical integration, industrial firms which integrated forward into marketing either bought out their distributors or created their own salaried sales force. The analogy to these developments would be the employment of a salaried physician staff. Several observers of hospital-based physician arrangements, including Dean Grant and Dr. George Criles, surgeon-in-chief of the Cleveland Clinic, believe that as physicians grow more plentiful, hospitals should use their market power to compel physicians to accept salaried arrangements in order to discourage abuse of the fee-for-service system. For many reasons, salaried employment of admitting physicians has not spread beyond the teaching and public/general hospitals. In community hospitals with teaching programs, typically only the director of medical education for the hospital or its various departments is likely to be salaried.

As mentioned above, physicians resent the institutionalization of medical practice and view it as a threat to their livelihoods. One physician complained that

> emergency department services are expanding into bases for conventional ambulatory care and . . . directors of special laboratories in the hospital are being encouraged to organize clinics or are offered practice privileges so that they might provide continuing care in certain subspecialty areas, thus competing with community based physicians in comparable specialty fields.[8]

Physicians may view their hospitals as a menancing combination of financial and technical power, dwarfing individual and group practices and threatening their economic viability.

Anxieties have led medical staffs to oppose the development of hospital-based outpatient departments and/or expansion of emergency facilities in hospitals. They have sometimes led to medical staff demands that hospital contracts with salaried physicians clearly specify that at the conclusion of their period of salaried employment the contracting physician may not establish a practice within so many miles of the hospital. These covenants may or may not be legally enforceable. In some teaching hospitals salaried attending physicians may be limited to admission of patients only through the emergency room, or to supervision of treatment by interns and residents on ward or charity services. These provisions assure that attending physicians' medical activities do not compete with the practices of voluntary admitting physicians.

Some industry observers have speculated that in high physician surplus areas hospital administrators will have sufficient bargaining power to increase the proportion of physicians on the medical staff who are employees of the hospital or which are under contractual arrangements which provide managerial control over physician practice. This issue will be discussed below.

CLOSURE OF MEDICAL STAFFS

Another area of potential conflict involves the control ceded most medical staffs by hospital bylaws over credentialing and the granting of hospital privileges to potential new members of the medical staff. This control is necessary for effective peer review and quality assurance activity in the hospital. But it raises another area of major potential conflict between physicians and hospital—medical staff closure.

In many instances, the closure of a medical staff may reflect some simple realities. The hospital may not be able to accomodate additional patients with the number of beds it is currently operating. To admit additional physicians to the medical staff in such a case would compromise the ability of existing physicians to get their patients into the house when they need to. In teaching hospital settings, medical staffs may be closed to assure that only those individuals with appropriate academic qualifications are granted privileges to practice and teach medicine in its programs.

But there are instances where closure of a medical staff may not be the result of a full hospital or a specialized mission. Some medical staffs may withhold privileges to discourage new physician competitors from entering the community or to deny "undesirable" physicians (of the "wrong" race, religion, or nationality) access to the facility. In some rural areas, and in many inner city areas as well, where the hospital is the only place to practice, such actions may be effective in keeping new physician competitors out of the communities, protecting established practices and incomes. In instances where the hospital is not full, or has declining occupancy, medical staff exercise of this power may put the hospital in an untenable position.

The issue of staff privileges is a vital one for the physician, both financially and professionally. Accordingly it has become a subject of increasing litigation and public controversy in some parts of the country with high concentrations of physicians. In New York City, for example, legislative hearings in 1971 established that some 30 percent of physicians in the New York City area lacked medical staff privileges at any hospital.* After confronting the lack of legal jurisdiction over the credentials and privileges functions of private hospitals, some legislators sought to prevent alleged discrimination by private hospitals by spelling out in state law concrete guidelines for granting privileges. The predictable result was the establishment of an appeals mechanism without enforcement power.[9]

Some legal scholars have speculated that the granting of staff privileges will become a major antitrust issue, since closing of medical staffs or exclusion of certain practitioners could be construed as an exercise of monopoly power. In a discussion of the anti-trust implications of medical staff privileges, a *Duke Law Journal* commentator established that courts have found that medical staff privileges are both a professional and financial necessity for the practicing physician and may be recognized by the courts as a property, as well as a personal, right.[10] Though there has been little

---

* Presumably this means that they must forego income related to hospitalizing their patients and refer them to physicians who do have such privileges.

litigation on this subject so far, the growing density of physicians in the United States suggests that this will be a fertile area for legal conflict between physicians and between the physician and the hospital.

As mentioned above, from the hospital standpoint the problem becomes critical when falling productivity, whether in the hospital as a whole or in individual departments, imperils the hospital's financial position or threatens the quality of care in the hospital. The ability of the administrator or trustees to intervene directly in such instances may depend on institutional politics more than formal exercise of power. While in the case of individual departments, the administrator may have leverage through the budget process in approving equipment or personnel requests or in making renovations or other capital expenditures, that person has almost no leverage with a united medical staff except to point out the economic consequenses of closure for the continued ability of the hospital to maintain efficient operations.

In instances where other hospitals in the community keep their staffs open, the closure of a medical staff may merely be a self-defeating gesture, compelling new physicians to practice at competing institutions. The threat to the livelihoods of the physicians in the community will continue but the hospital with a closed staff will simply be deprived of the marginal income. The ineffectiveness and ultimately self-defeating nature of such a partial measure should be publicly apparent, hence easier to defuse.

PHYSICIAN RECRUITMENT

A related though less acute problem involves recruitment of physicians to the medical staff and the community. Members of the community and the hospital administrator may agree that more physicians are needed in the community. Such a conclusion may be drawn from a careful analysis of the productivity or age structure of the hospital's medical staff, or a growing number of patients with no physician crowding a facility's emergency room, or the pending retirement of one or more key admitters to the hospital. However, the perceived need for additional practitioners in the community may not be shared by members of the medical staff.

The lack of a sufficiently active or committed medical staff, or the impending departure of key admitters, threatens the hospital's financial viability. Yet the decision to intervene in physician recruitment inevitably trespasses on what the community physician may consider to be his or her economic turf. Physicians are intensely territorial. Their anxieties about additional physician competition in their community may reflect not hard economic reality so much as a fear of the unknown. Similarly, inquiries by hospital administrators or trustees about a physician's retirement plans may be viewed as an unwarranted intrusion into the physician's private sphere.

Legitimation of the hospital's concerns about the productivity of the medical staff and the community's concern about adequate physician coverage is the central task in physician recruitment. Having an adequate data base is a key factor in legitimating the concern. It is also important for physicians to understand that the availability of resources to meet their needs both for equipment and staff, as well as modern facilities, may be linked to physician activity which guarantees a net income for the hospital. Administrators who fail to involve key representatives of the medical staff and community in recruitment may experience significant political difficulties.

STRATEGIC CONCERNS IN RESOLVING MD-HOSPITAL ECONOMIC CONFLICT

It should be clear from the foregoing discussion that the physician and the hospital are economically interdependent. Yet the areas of divergence of economic interest present a difficult and potentially explosive managerial problem. Tightening competitive markets both for hospitals and physicians will create fertile ground for potential conflict between the physician and the hospital. Those who seek conflict from either side are likely to find it. If this conflict is aggravated both parties lose, and the patient loses, perhaps more.

Some observers of the physician-hospital relationship, such as Dean Grant, believe with some passion that the hospital has a social, even a moral, responsibility to compel physicians to accept contractual arrangements with the hospital which subject their activities to managerial oversight. This view argues that since the hospital is responsible for granting monopoly power to its hospital-based physicians and franchises for hospital practice to its admitters, it should bear the responsibility for preventing their abuse of economic power. Implicit in Grant's view is that physician incomes for hospital-based practitioners, in particular, are too high, and that permitting unreasonable incomes damages the hospital's legitimacy in the community.

At the same time, many hospital planners believe that the hospital's objective of maintaining its utilization override the particular short-run interests of the medical staff in protecting their individual practices. Apocryphal tales circulate in some planning circles about hospital management companies so powerful that, to preserve their hospitals, they can afford to "fire" their medical staffs over costs issues and recruit new ones from around the country. A hospital-centered approach to planning frequently produces large-scale hospital based ambulatory care centers and aggressive development of captive, satellite facilities staffed by salaried physicians.

Necessarily, an approach to resolving the inherent economic conflict between physician and hospital requires an admixture of values and prejudices. The approach below includes several:

1. The economic, social, and medical benefits of cooperation between administrators and physicians far outweigh the benefits accruing from conflict.
2. Physicians and administrators should seek to exploit their unique professional and managerial competences to assure an economically viable hospital in which quality patient care is practiced.
3. Physicians and administrators should avoid unreasonable intrusion into the areas of competence of the other.

There are many who believe that pursuing these values is impossible. Those individuals are likely to believe as well that the specific policy consequences of them are not achievable for that reason. There are many circumstances where historical practices or current institutional politics simply prevent them from being pursued. This, however, should not prevent them from being considered.

HOSPITAL OVERSIGHT OVER PHYSICIAN COMPENSATION

The primary responsibility of hospital administrators in relation to the physician is to assure efficient, cost-effective hospital operations. Since the institution is liable for instances of malpractice, they must concern themselves as well with the quality of care in their institutions. As a general principle, however, the hospital administrator, should not assume responsibility for oversight over the compensation of the physician. Neither administrators nor trustees possess a sufficiently objective basis for determining what equitable physician compensation ought to be. Neither do they have an objective method for determining the medical necessity of procedures prescribed for the patient's treatment. While the administrator should make sure that the facility is not being used in a way which violates the law, administrative responsibility for regulating the flow of income to the physician should stop there.

This does not mean that the administrator should abdicate professional responsibility for assuring the effective management of hospital departments. To the maximum extent possible, that person should strive to retain administrative control over hospital personnel and resources through salaried department managers. Furthermore, the administrator should insist on standards for purchase of equipment and commitment of additional personnel as rigorous in ancillary departments as in any other area of the hospital. Physicians should accept a data based framework for assessing capital and personnel needs as part of the managerial function of the hospital. This approach will become much more acceptable when it is clear to all parties that resources for patient care truly are limited.

The ultimate responsibility for preventing abuse of the economic power of the physician ultimately rests with the legal system and with those actors who pay for care—the third-party payer. These efforts are likely to intensify as resources for the health care field tighten. But the proximate responsibility for assuring that the power of the physician is not abused rests with the profession itself. While many medical societies have been reluctant to expel or discipline members who have engaged in medical profiteering or abuse, it is difficult to conceive of a system where effective medical judgment can be exercised by nonphysicians. If physicians choose to abdicate the responsibility for regulating themselves, they cannot legitimate their continued economic freedom and will not be permitted to keep it.

In some instances, obviously, disinterest in physician compensation is impossible. Teaching hospitals, government health care facilities, health maintenance organizations, private clinics like Mayo and the Cleveland Clinic—all these facilities have accomodated to salaried medical practice. For them, managerial responsibility for physician compensation is unavoidable. But even these organizations may reach fiscal limits which compel them to begin shifting some of the burden of physician compensation back onto the clinical marketplace and, implicitly, onto the physician. Hospital revenues are unlikely to grow sufficiently rapidly to sustain pure salary arrangements, and those institutions which have not developed incentive systems which involve some linkage between physician productivity and compensation will probably do so in the future.

As to the possibility that impending conditions of physician oversupply may create a buyers' market for physicians service, permitting hospitals to put more physicians "under contract," hospital resource constraints may not permit it. Hospitals have been under increasing pressure, from Medicare routine costs limits to rate review. This pressure will intensify if, as it appears likely, government begins to tighten Medicaid and Medicare spending. Pressures will intensify ever further under increased economic competition based upon price. Effective financial strategy involves managing the base of expenses in such a way that the hospital avoids financial responsibility for costs which are difficult to control. Hospital-based physician salary expenses are likely to be far more difficult to control than, say, janitorial expenses. Administrators will think twice before adding physician salary costs to their budgets in an increasingly resource-constrained environment.

Hospital administrators face so many battles in the heavily regulated, conflict-ridden environment that it becomes important to pick the ones that can be won. Winning a battle with a physician group over compensation is frequently a Pyrrhic victory and is likely to dissipate sufficient energy and legitimacy that the struggle will not only weaken the administrator but the institution as well. There are circumstances where such conflicts are not chosen, but inherited, and may be unavoidable. In these cases, it is usually essential to move quickly and to take no prisoners. But to the extent possible, hospital administrators should support the fee-for-service method of compensating physicians and strive to involve themselves as little as humanly and legally possible in physician compensation matters.

HOSPITAL COMPETITION WITH PHYSICIAN PRACTICE

As mentioned in the discussion of ambulatory care, hospitals which integrate forward into direct delivery of ambulatory care may put the hospital into conflict with the private practices of their medical staffs. In industry, however, forward integration did not occur unless it was possible to achieve efficiency and economies of scale which contributed to profit. If it cost more to create one's own sales force, transportation system, and so on than it did to take advantage of existing systems and intermediaries, manufacturing organizations retained the old system and confined their efforts to manufacturing.

In light of this observation, it is far from clear that hospital-based outpatient medical practice is a cost-effective alternative to office based practice. Figure 8–2 illustrates the comparative costs of a visit to a large urban hospital and a visit to a group practice in the Chicago area. A hospital outpatient visit costs fully triple that of comparable service in a group practice setting. This disparity is representative of the relative costs of practice in the two settings. The cost structure of hospital outpatient visits is dictated largely by the reimbursement practices of Medicare and Medicaid, which require allocation of full hospital overheads to outpatient cost centers. Charges for physicians office visits are not subject to such overhead allocations. The physician's fee covers overhead costs, which are much lower than the hospital's.

FIGURE 8–2
Comparative cost structure: group practices and hospital outpatient clinics

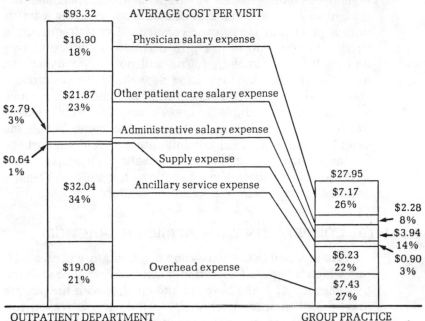

$93.32   AVERAGE COST PER VISIT

$16.90   Physician salary expense
18%

$21.87   Other patient care salary expense
23%

$2.79
3%

Administrative salary expense

$0.64   Supply expense
1%

$27.95

$32.04   Ancillary service expense
34%

$7.17 $2.28
26%   ← 8%

←$3.94
14%

$6.23 $0.90
22%   3%

$19.08   Overhead expense
21%

$7.43
27%

OUTPATIENT DEPARTMENT   GROUP PRACTICE

Source: Reprinted by permission Booz, Allen & Hamilton.

Physician practices are more likely to substitute technicians for ancillary physicians (radiologists and pathologists) and are less likely to have unionized clerical or technical staff.

Medicare principles further dictate that a hospital's charges must be reasonably related to cost and that Medicare will pay the lower of cost or charges, in the aggregate. In practice this means that one must charge the non-Medicare patient at least as much as one charges the government for caring for the elderly. The concern about not subsidizing private care to the wealthy with public funds is certainly appropriate. In practice however, when combined with over-head allocation requirements, the "lower of cost or charges" provision means that hospitals cannot price their outpatient services competitively. Furthermore, because the absolute level of charges has become so high, and because of skimpy health insurance coverage of outpatient costs, outpatient care produces enough bad debts to render it a money losing operation.

Some facilities, notably Massachusetts General Hospital, have been able to create the proper mixture of physician incentives and cost controls to make the hospital-based outpatient clinic work. But it is a losing battle. Hospital outpatient departments are costly dinosaurs. Rather than encourage additional outpatient coverage or reallocate costs to encourage more competitive rates, the U.S. Senate passed legislation in 1980 to establish routine costs limits for outpatient care, heretofore not subject to such limits. In Illinois, the Medicaid hospital outpatient reimbursement for some hospitals has reached a level of 10 times the reimbursement for a basic physician's office visit. This cannot long endure.*

As if the cost problems were not enough, hospital capital expenditures for outpatient facilities, including satellites, were brought under Certificate of Need in the 1977 amendments to the Federal Health Planning Act. This means not only that hospitals contemplating construction of such facilities can anticipate lengthy delays (of up to two years from commencement of planning to approval of the CoN) but they expose themselves to the wrath of competing facilities and physicians in public hearings.

If it were possible for hospitals to provide on-site outpatient care of a higher quality than that available in the community, it might be worth the fight. But progressive health care institutions, such as Rush Presbyterian-St. Lukes Medical Center and Mt. Sinai Hospital in Chicago were able to develop alternative structures which both provided the amenities of physician practice and lower cost to the patient, and got out of the hospital-based outpatient business altogether. Over the next 10 to 15 years many large hospitals may begin to move in the same direction, though the toal shutdown accomplished by Rush in 1974 may no longer be feasible. It does not make medical or financial sense for the hospital to compete with its physicians in the ambulatory care sector, particularly if its objectives can be achieved through a cooperative approach.

---

* Indeed, as this book was being edited, the Illinois Medicaid agency proposed to implement sharp, unilateral reductions in hospital-based outpatient reimbursement, which may severely damage Chicago's teaching hospitals.

SUPPORT OF PHYSICIAN PRACTICE

It should be clear from the foregoing discussion that hospital-based ambulatory programs may not be cost-effective feeder systems. As the Rush system demonstrated, however, there are a variety of alternatives to hospital-based facilities which can accomplish the same objective. Large hospitals have the capital resources to develop physicians' office buildings or community-based ambulatory programs.

However, even the small hospital has an enormous technical and organizational advantage over the largest group practice in evaluating and initiating new ventures in primary care. Compared to the hospital, a medical practice is a thinly capitalized, undermanaged, relatively fragile enterprise. As hospitals have staffed up to cope with the legal, regulatory, and financial problems they face, they have accumulated expertise which can, under appropriate circumstances, be of enormous assistance to the practicing physicians on the hospital's medical staff.

Hospitals have legal counsel, reimbursement specialists, facilities planners, purchasing agents, community liaisons, and marketing specialists on their staffs. Through contractual relationships, hospitals have access to accounting and specialized legal expertise, as well as to consulting assistance. Their boards of trustees frequently contain banking and financial leaders as well as individuals who invest venture capital. In short, hospitals are reservoirs of expertise and can tap external financial resources which under some circumstances may not be available to the physician coping with new practice opportunities and increasing competition.

Hospitals should consider making these technical and financial resources available on a joint venture basis to selected members of their medical staffs to further their professional practices or to permit them to develop new forms of health care delivery. Hospital planners can be of enormous assistance in identifying new practice opportunities—areas in the community that lack a sufficient number of physicians or that lack certain ambulatory medical services. Hospital attorneys and reimbursement specialists can help devise charge structures that will maximize income as well as help avoid billing practices which may compromise the physician legally. Outside counsel and accountants can help (particularly the new) physician develop a corporate structure for physician practice which maximizes income as well as personal financial plans for the physician. Hospital trustees and their colleagues in the community can help arrange financing for medical office buildings, and facilities planners can help assure efficient design and construction.

This approach is not without significant legal and political problems. If done on a large scale, hospital technical assistance to individual physicians, or to physician groups, could be viewed by the Internal Revenue Service (which has become increasingly active in health care matters) as "innurement of benefits" to specific individuals, thus jeopardizing the hospital's tax-exempt status. The not-for-profit status granted under Section 501 (c) (3) of the federal tax code is predicated upon the fact that the benefits of the organization will not innure to individuals—that it cannot profit individual practitioners, administrators, or trustees. This problem can be avoided by discretion, or by nominal charges for the consulting services of the hospital's technical staff.

If, on the other hand, such services are arranged through formal contracts which bind the physician to bring patients to the facility providing the assistance, the contracts could be interpreted as violating the same antifraud provisions of Medicare and Medicaid that forbid such practices as fee-splitting. The same is true of explicit language in agreements concerning physician recruitment, a legal problem which, if foreseen, can be avoided. The hospital should not be construed as offering its resources in exchange for physician business through formal contracts. It is far better to offer types of assistance which, if withdrawn, pose some economic risk to the physician, and to let the performance expected under terms of such an agreement remain implicit, though crystal clear. If physicians are using hospital office space or facilities, but are hospitalizing their patients at a competing institution, it is clearly justifiable for the administrator to refuse to renew the physicians' lease.

A stickier problem with the joint venture approach discussed above is one of equity. That is, how can the administrator or trustees of a hospital justify rendering assistance to some but not all members of a medical staff? The problem is partially political and merits a partially political answer. Hospital resources should be devoted, to the extent practical, to further the interests of those who support the hospital. Not all physicians make an equal contribution to the vitality of the hospital—every facility has a group of key admitters who are loyal to the hospital. It is these individuals, and the younger colleagues who will be recruited onto the staff, who will become tomorrow's key admitters, who merit the hospital's assistance. Effective administrators have always found ways of rewarding those who keep the hospital solvent. In the past this involved allocations of resources from the hospital budget, on the margin. In the future the ability to reward performance through purchasing equipment or adding nursing staff will be compromised by cost containment. Thus administrators must think more creatively about how to signal their appreciation for the loyalty of their physicians. Joint ventures and hospital technical assistance are powerful tools for use in the appropriate climate.

Hospitals have a compelling economic interest in the health and welfare of their physicians. Their practices are the primary feeder system for the hospital and the success their physicians have in penetrating and holding a share of the physician marketplace will have a direct bearing on the utilization of the hospital. *Hospitals do not need to own or operate their own feeder systems.* Through joint ventures, they can assure the same result—sustained hospital utilization—by assuring that their medical staffs have the resources to practice competitive medicine. Since physicians are not subject to Certificate of Need laws, facilities they construct and equipment they acquire are not subject to the delays, public exposure, and bureaucratic harrassment to which hospitals are subjected. Physicians can act quickly and without regulatory oversight to do the very same things which would take hospitals, in some cases, years of effort and politics to accomplish. The freedom of the physician can be turned to the advantage of those hospitals who recognize the opportunities inherent in that freedom.

There is no good reason for the hospital to hoard the considerable technical and financial expertise it has accumulated. On the contrary, by making these resources available to the core of physicians who are loyal to the hospital, those resources can be put to work outside the hospital to further its corporate objectives. Hospitals need not intrude into the physician practice sphere if it is clear they are neither needed or wanted. But they should be prepared to broaden access to their technical and external financial resources if the climate of cooperation and interest on the part of physicians exists. Hospitals and physicians should be allies in the increasingly competitive health care market, and should strive to maximize their respective competitive advantages.

NOTES

1. Jon R. Gabel and Michael A. Redisch, "Alternative Physician Payment Methods: Incentives, Efficiency, and National Health Insurance," *Milbank Memorial Fund Quarterly/Health and Society,* 57, no. 1 (1979): 38.
2. Dean Grant, *How to Negotiate Physician Contracts* (Chicago: Teach 'em Inc. 1979), p. 110.
3. Bruce Steinwald, "Hospital Based Physicians Current Issues and Descriptive Evidence," *Health Care Financing Review,* (Summer 1980), p. 73.
4. Ibid., p. 72.
5. James A. Morell and Peter G. Rogan, "Hospital Based Physician Compensation Concepts," *Topics in Health Care Financing,* "Physician Compensation," ed. David Pieroni, (Spring 1978), p. 17.
6. Ibid., p. 18.
7. Ibid., p. 17.
8. Roy Perkins, M.D. "The Physicians' View of the Hospital: A Love-Hate Relationship," *The Hospital Medical Staff: Selected Readings 1972–1978* (Chicago: American Hospital Association, 1977), p. 113.
9. "Physician-Hospital Conflict: The Hospital Staff Privileges Controversy in New York," *Cornell Law Review* 60 (1975):1097.
10. "Physician Influence: Applying Noerr-Pennington to the Medical Profession," *Duke Law Journal* 19 (May 1978):715.

9 The crisis in nursing: Implications for the hospital

Nurses are as essential to most forms of organized health care as gasoline is to automobiles. The adequacy of supply of nurses to the health care industry is not only essential to its ongoing operation, but critical to institutions which attempt to diversify into new forms of care, many of which are nursing-intensive. It is ironic that facilities and professionals which have succeeded in developing competitive strategies for attracting patients may founder in their inability to attract and retain sufficient nurses to treat them. A major bottleneck in securing adequate nursing "person-power" is emerging in the United States, one which may compromise the quality of patient care and inhibit the evolution of new forms of health care.

The surface manifestation of the nursing crisis has been a growing gap between nurse staffing requirements of hospitals, nursing homes, and other institutional providers and the number of nurses in the labor market. Underlying the shortage of nurses, however, is a deeper crisis of a profession seeking to redefine its role in a changing health care system.

Understanding the nature and origins of this crisis is an essential precondition of developing a strategy to deal with it. The nursing crisis presents health care providers with a marketing problem of a different sort and is forcing professionals and managers to understand better the needs and aspirations of nurses.

EVIDENCE OF THE PROBLEM

The increasing difficulty which health care institutions have encountered in recruiting and retaining nurses began to attract national attention during 1979 and 1980. Articles in national news magazines and in local newspapers began to document the struggles of hospitals and nursing homes in securing sufficient nurses. Hospitals have reported closing down beds and intensive care units in some parts of the country, and embarking on aggressive recruiting campaigns involving national advertising, enhanced fringe benefits, and wage differentials.[1] These are the manifestations of a classic labor shortage.

Hospital industry sources have estimated that the current shortage of registered nurses (RNs) in the industry approaches 100,000 persons.[2] Spokespersons for the National League of Nursing estimated that the shortage in the nursing home industry is even larger, approximately 150,000 vacant positions for RNs and nurses at lower skill levels.[3] Data on shortages in public health clinics, schools, and physicians' offices are not readily available.

Several groups have attempted to gather more detailed information on the extent of the shortage nationwide. Early in 1980 the National Association of Nurse Recruiters (NANR) polled its membership on the extent of their nursing vacancies. The institutions that responded to the survey reported an average of 72.5 vacant RN positions per hospital.[4] There were significant regional differences in vacancies, with southern and western hospitals reporting the largest problems. Hospitals responding to the survey reported an average annual nursing turnover rate of 32 percent, with highest vacancy rates in medical/surgical and intensive care positions.

Another national survey was conducted by *RN Magazine* during the same period.[5] This survey found that 88 percent of the hospitals which responded had nursing vacancies and 90 percent of the respondents characterized the supply problem as serious. Fully one half of the respondents reported intensive care nursing vacancies and 42 percent, medical/surgical vacancies. The average annual turnover rate for nursing positions was 29 percent, reasonably close to the NANR results. While only 34 percent of the hospitals reported difficulties in filling part-time positions, 96 percent reported difficulty in filling full-time positions. As with the NANR survey, hospitals in the southern and western parts of the country reported the greatest difficulties.

Both surveys had relatively small samples, skewed toward larger hospitals. Because of the skew toward facilities which may have better organized or better financed nurse recruitment efforts, the data may actually underestimate the extent of the problem.

In Illinois, an Illinois Hospital Association survey conducted during January 1980 covered 92 percent of the state's 259 hospitals.[6] This survey documented a 12.5 percent vacancy rate for RNs in Illinois hospitals, which translated into 5,321 vacant positions. The vast majority of these vacancies were in staff RN positions. There was also a 12.1 percent shortfall of the staff LPN (licensed practical nurse), a lower-skilled nurse, which translated into 1,365 unfilled positions. The total nursing shortfall in Illinois hospitals was 7,830 positions, compared to 73,592 budgeted positions.

As a result of these shortages, 48 Illinois hospitals, 20 percent of those reporting, experienced temporary or permanent bed closures during the previous year. These closures involved 891 beds, or 1.5 percent of the total bed complement of reporting institutions. Of these beds 140, or 26 percent, were in intensive care units, while 636 were in medical/surgical units.

Hospital administrators in the East and Midwest have speculated that their nurse staffing problems are created in part by migration of nurses to warmer, more attractive climates. The data does not bear out this contention. On the contrary, California, which has sustained immigration from a number of occupational groups for many years, has one of the most serious nursing shortage problems of anywhere in the country, one which appeared to worsen during the late 1970s. The California Hospital Association reported that budgeted but unfilled RN positions climbed from 14 percent in 1977 to 20 percent in the first half of 1979. Most of the vacancies are reported in night shifts (43 percent), with rural hospitals experiencing especially serious difficulty.[7]

Labor force participation by nurses

Despite these demonstrably serious problems, in justifying denials of federal assistance for training more nurses, federal budget officials have insisted that there are plenty of nurses in the United States already. How can this be? Simple enough—the rate of *labor force participation* among licensed RNs is not sufficient to meet the growing demand for their services. During 1977 a joint study by the Department of Health and Human Services (HHS) and American Nursing Association study estimated that there were approximately 1.4 million registered nurses in the United States capable of working as nurses. Yet only about 70 percent, or about 988,000, were actually working. Of this number, only 60 percent were employed full-time. Thus, only 42 percent of the RNs in the United States were employed full-time in their profession.[8] The National League of Nursing puts the labor force participation rate of nurses even lower than ANA estimates, at around 60 percent.

Labor force participation of RNs drops sharply in the first five years after graduation from nursing education programs. If one examines nursing career patterns, it can be seen that between the first and fifth year after baccalaureate the percentage of nurses working full-time drops from 84.5 percent to 46.7 percent, while the percentage not working increases from 10.1 to 36.5. The shift from full-time to part-time nursing employment is a longer term phenomenon, increasing from 4.6 percent a year after graduation to 14.6 percent after five years, to 22.1 percent after 10 years.[9]

This pattern of labor force participation is not dissimilar to those of teachers and social workers, roles filled traditionally by women. The same HHS/ANA study estimated that only 1.9 percent of all licensed registered nurses in 1977 were men, compared to 1.3 percent in 1972.[10] In contrast to nursing, however, the demand for teachers and social workers has lessened markedly in recent years. There is some evidence that family obligations play a significant role in the pattern, for example, that nurses drop out of the full-time labor market to raise children and reenter at the part-time level when their children reach school age. However, survey data which will be discussed below suggest that family obligations are not the primary reason for the low rate of labor force participation among registered nurses.

Outlook for the balance of supply and demand for nurses

Impending developments both on the supply and demand side of the equation render the future nursing outlook extremely bleak for health care providers. On the supply side, the demographic trends for the 1980s and 1990s forecast a sharply diminishing pool of young people from which entrants into the nursing profession will be drawn. Furthermore, enrollment in nursing schools peaked in the mid-1970s. According to the National League of Nursing, the number of first-year students admitted to nursing degree programs declined nearly 3 percent from 1977 to 1979, while total enrollment in RN programs declined in 1979 for the fourth year in a row. The 1 percent decline in graduates of such programs from 1978 to 1979 was the first since the mid-1960s.[11] Though new baccalaureate nursing programs continue to be added to university curricula, hospital-based diploma programs, which provided large numbers of grass roots nursing personnel, continue to close under continued hospital cost pressure. Those who look to increasing production of nurses to alleviate the shortage will find no relief in the forseeable future.

On the other side, estimates of growth in nursing demand vary. A 1978 analysis conducted by the Western Interstate Commission for Higher Education (WICHE) projected 1982 RN requirements nationwide at between 1.2 and 1.6 million full-time equivalent positions. The growth in hospital demand for nursing personnel was projected at between 84 and 137 percent between 1976 (the study's base year) and 1982. Demand for nursing personnel in the nursing home industry was projected to increase by from 174 to 466 percent during the same six-year period. Substantial demand increases were also forecast for community, school, and occupational health facilities, as well as more modest increases in demand at the physicians' office level.[12] The Department of Health, and Human Services predicted demanded by 1985 at the only slightly more conservative level of between 1.2 and 1.3 million, or between 20 and 30 percent more nurses than were in the labor market in 1977.[13]

Figure 9–1 shows the distribution of nurses among various health care providers according to the 1977 HEW/ANA national survey. According to the study, the sectors where demand grew fastest during the period 1972–77 were in the public/community health areas and in the nursing home and extended care areas. As established earlier, there was substantial expansion of both sectors in the late 1960s and in the nursing home industry in the early 1970s. Data on

FIGURE 9–1
Where are RNs working

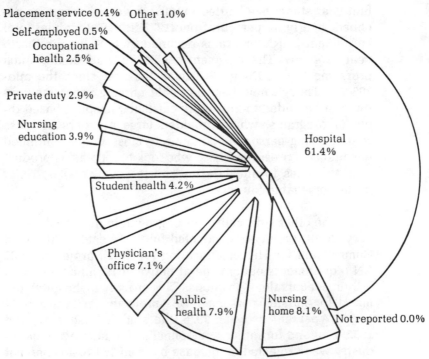

Source: American Journal of Nursing, October 1979.

nursing career patterns suggest that there is considerable nurse mobility between providers. Specifically, the share of nursing positions claimed by hospitals declines from 66 percent a year after graduation to 42 percent after 10 years. The chief beneficiaries of this shift were nursing schools, which claimed a 15 percent share 10 years out, community health agencies, with 10 percent, and schools with 6 percent.[14]

Growing demand in the hospital field has stemmed not so much from a growth in the number of facilities as from an increase in complexity, both organizational and technological. Specialization within clinical medicine has led to parallel specialization in the nursing field, in such areas as emergency medicine, intensive care, and geriatric medicine. Growth in supply of nursing specialists has lagged considerably behind the growth in the facilities and programs they serve.

Concepts such as primary nursing have also made hospitals increasingly nursing-intensive. Primary nursing is conceptually simple but organizationally complex. The core concept is that each patient is to identify with a *single nurse* as having responsibility for the continuity of patient care. The rationale for the concept is compelling: both patients and nurses find the team nursing approach, with multiple layers of accountability and a shifting cast of characters, alienating and unsatisfactory.

In theory, primary nursing reduced the patient load while still providing the nurse with nursing assistant support for technical problems.[15] In addition to providing a more satisfying nursing role in patient management, the implementation of primary nursing helped solve a problem of underutilized nursing assistants (by using fewer of them). The price for these improvements is a more RN-intensive staffing pattern and a greater demand for scarce RNs in the hospital. Nursing supply problems may necessitate abandonment of the pure form of primary nursing and compel some accommodation with team nursing. The hybrid staffing pattern has become known as modular nursing, a system which may be more sparing of RN resources, yet retaining the concept of RN responsibility for a limited panel of patients.

CAUSES OF THE CRISIS

There is a lot of speculation in the health care industry about why it is unable to attract and retain a sufficient supply of competent nurses. It is difficult to answer the question definitively without thinking about the role of the nurse in the health care system. The nurse is responsible for the continuity and progress of organized patient care. Where that care is imbedded in a bureaucratic setting, the nurse has pivotal responsibility for assembling and focussing institutional resources on the patient's problem. In settings where directives from the physician are ambiguous, or the support systems which are supposed to provide the resources (supplies and services) for patient care break down, or more to the point of the supply crisis, where nursing staffing is stretch thin, nursing becomes an almost impossible struggle.

Health care organizations themselves are complex, and lines of authority cross and conflict in many cases. Requirements for financial accountability in hospitals have escalated to the point where bureaucratic systems have almost overwhelmed the core patient care mission of the physician and nurse. Hospitals, in particular, have become mazes of information and control systems whose mandates and data requirements seem almost completely arbitrary to those rendering patient care.

All the pressures generated by these systems force their way into the nursing routine. The results of this process are not pleasant. Terms like *burnout* and *reality shock* creep into the vocabulary of analysis of the problem. These stress factors associated with delivery of organized patient care are among the highest in the U.S. occupational system. Hospitals in particular offer high-stress environments. When the National Institute for Occupational Safety and Health (NIOSH) studied the relative incidence of mental disorders in 130 occupational groups, 7 of the top 27 occupations related to health care. Further, studies have linked high-stress occupations to high on-the-job and off-the-job accident rates.[16] Manifestations of high-stress occupations in the workplace include lower productivity, high turnover, absenteeism, increased work errors, and other factors.

All these features impinge on the nurse in a hospital setting and affect ability to function effectively. In a survey of nurses who dropped out of the profession, the bureaucracy and its demands are cited as the principal cause of decisions to leave, far outranking low wages. "Increased demands resulting in lack of patient contact" were cited by 35 percent of the dropouts in an industry survey, outranking "family related problems," cited by 31 percent, and "low wages," cited by only 13 percent.[17]

Of those nurses surveyed who were working as nurses, only 10.8 percent indicated that they were very satisfied with their work. In ranking problems they considered to be crucial, the bureaucratic setting emerged near the head of the list. Among working nurses, 55.6 percent complained about having "no input on matters concerning them," 49.4 percent of "excessive demands on them," and 41 percent of "too much paperwork." "Low patient care standards" were listed by 55.1 percent and "not enough say in patient care" by 43.3 percent.[18]

Though wages are not the foremost cause of disillusionment, they remain a significant problem. The nursing profession has the unusual feature of an almost flat wage curve relative to experience. In hospital-to-hospital job movement, nearly all mobility is "lateral." Only one nurse in five surveyed reported upward mobility professionally as a result of a job move.[19] In a survey by *RN Magazine,* more than half of those nurses with 15 or more years of experience reported that they earn in the same range ($5 to $7.50 an hour) that 79 percent of new graduates in nursing are earning after less than a year.[20] Even nurses with advanced degrees do not appear to be significantly rewarded. See Figure 9–2.

The implication of this state of affairs is that, at least from a wage standpoint, seniority and education are not rewarded economically. Even moving into a shortage speciality like intensive care is, surprisingly, not economically rewarding. There is almost no spread between short-supply specialties and specialties where there is adequate supply. Furthermore, RNs with specialty certification make only about $800 per year more than the average generalist RN. There are virtually no financial incentives to fill specialty areas which are short, and none to remain in the profession for a lengthy period of time. See Figure 9–3.

FIGURE 9–2
How degrees affect your income

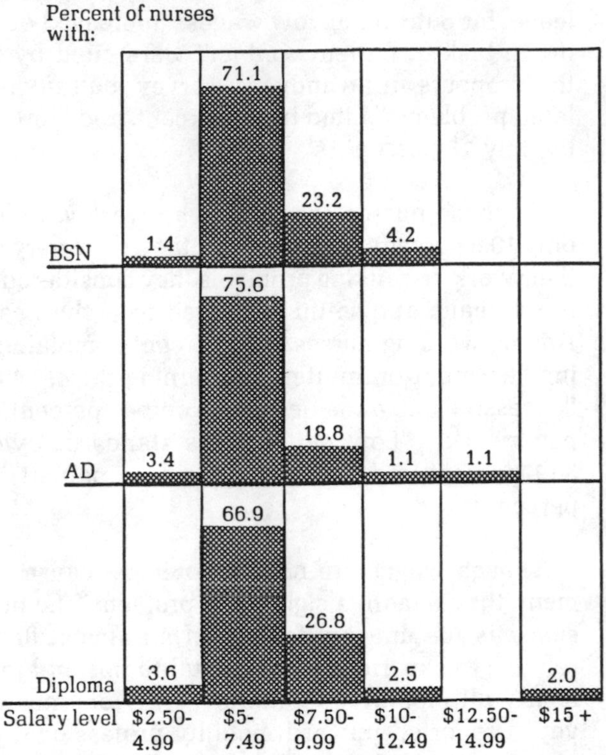

Percent of nurses
with:

Salary level	$2.50-4.99	$5-7.49	$7.50-9.99	$10-12.49	$12.50-14.99	$15 +
BSN	1.4	71.1	23.2	4.2		
AD	3.4	75.6	18.8	1.1	1.1	
Diploma	3.6	66.9	26.8	2.5		2.0

Source: *RN Magazine*, February 1980.

However, the most serious problem underlying the "churning" occupational pattern of nurses may be the mismatch of expectations generated during nursing education and the reality of the nursing role. Humanistic and intellectual values play a large role in the decision to enter nursing. Nursing education tends to reinforce these values as it becomes increasingly important in defining the profession's "self image." At the same time, nursing education programs are becoming increasingly rigorous and demanding intellectually, particularly respecting academic requirements. Many nursing degree programs at the bachelors' level require much basic and biological science course work, while masters programs may require formal theses. Many of those who train in these programs may be unequipped motivationally to play the multiple roles of clerk, supply sergeant, transportation

FIGURE 9–3
Which services pay best

Service	Mean hourly earnings
Geriatrics	$6.40
Pediatrics	$6.77
Orthopedics	$6.86
Medical/surgical	$6.85
Cardiac care unit	$6.87
Newborn	$6.96
Emergency room	$6.99
Intensive care unit	$7.07
Obstetrics/gynecology	$7.08
Outpatient	$7.14
Operating room	$8.19*
Psychiatry	$8.41*

* Estimated hourly earnings based on reported mean annual salary.
Source: *RN Magazine.* February 1980.

aide, and unit manager which have, in some settings, grafted themselves onto the core patient care function of the nurse. Nurses also do not accommodate easily to the attitudes of many physicians who view them as little more than manual laborers in white uniforms.

Perhaps the most difficult adjustment of all, however, is to the hospital's status hierarchy. Advancement and status is keyed to increasing administrative responsibility. This responsibility, particularly in larger hospitals, moves the nurse farther away from patient care until that function disappears from the job description. Thus nurses are often forced to choose among status, advancement and the higher pay associated with administrative responsibilities, and the values that motivated them to become nurses in the first place. As some critics of the nursing work role put it, "the nursing variation of the 'Peter Principle'. . . takes effective clinicians and makes them into mediocre bureaucrats, leaving only less experienced nurses to actually perform patient care functions."[21]

Job dissatisfaction is the principal result of disparity between career image and nursing reality. While 92 percent of nurses surveyed in a recent study named a "sense of achievement" as a very important factor in their work, only 32.7 percent felt "very satisfied" with the way their present

job met that need. While 76.5 percent cited "intellectual stim-
ulation" as a very important career factor, only 28 percent
were satisfied with this aspect of their current work. While
90 percent felt that "knowing that you help others" was a
very important career objective, only a little more than half
(55.1 percent) felt their current job satisfied them.[22] That
many nurses seem unable to derive intellectual and personal
satisfactions from the work environment poses the most serious challenge of all to those who employ nurses.

SUPPLEMENTAL NURSING AND STAFFING REQUIREMENTS

In more plentiful times hospitals coped with the variability
of nurse staffing needs in two ways—the use of overtime
pay and the development of a "float pool" of nurses without
specific unit assignments. As financial stringency and shortages have developed, overtime pay is now subject to ration-
ing and float pools are not adequate to meet shifting staffing
needs. The float positions themselves are low status, difficult
to fill and far from satisfying as nursing experience.

The result of the growing mismatch between available
nurses and nurse staffing needs has been the creation of
an entrepreneurial sector of supplemental nurse staffing
agencies, or nursing registries. Supplemental staffing agencies have played a major role in clerical/secretarial and day
labor markets for some time, but their appearance in the
nursing field is a product of the growing nurse staffing problems of the 1970s. Nurse registries retain nurses on an hourly
basis and tailor work hours to the particular requirements
of their nurses. The registries are low overhead operations
and, beyond social security, provide a stripped-down package of benefits to all but the longest-term nurse participants.[23]

Since the registries have positioned themselves as an alternative to overtime, the charge to the hospital, while lower
than overtime pay, is frequently substantially above conventional nurse expense levels for the hospital (as much as 30
percent higher in some cases). In 1980 in Illinois, the average
per shift cost of an RN from a registry was almost $97![24]
Nursing registries have flourished in high shortage areas.
In Illinois, 32 percent of hospitals participating in the Illinois
Hospital Association survey of nursing vacancies reported

using registries. Funds paid to the registries by these hospitals in 1979 totalled $23.6 million. In the Chicago area, however, 68 percent of the hospitals reporting using registries, double the statewide percentage.[25] No data was available on the relative productivity of registry nurses from the study.

While the registries meet some hospital needs for which adequate provision cannot always be made (coverage of vacation and sick leave), both nursing professionals and hospital administrators are uncomfortable about the cost and quality of care implications of increasing reliance on the registries for routine staffing needs. Temporary nurses have no institutional allegiance, though they may elect to work in a single or a few institutions, and are unlikely to contribute to team building or to morale. Staff nurses and physicians are sometimes hostile to temporary personnel and question their commitment to nursing.

Obviously, the learning curve for a temporary nurse is extremely steep, and the hospital reaps no benefits of increased productivity from the nurse's period of service in the institution. Some hospital industry representatives have urged the incorporation of an index of intensity of use of supplemental agencies (as a percentage of FTE nurse staffing) as a hospital accreditation criterion. Research on the connection between reliance on supplemental nurses and the quality of patient care may be a necessary prerequisite of such a development.

But to the extent that the registries meet the needs of the *nurse*, particularly for flexibility of work assignment, shift, and duty, the hospital, and for that matter other health care providers, will be forced to compete with the registries for nursing personnel in the future. This competition will intensify as the shortage grows and as registries develop marketing expertise to fine-tune pricing, recruitment, strategy, benefit packages, and other items to match to the growing expertise of institutional providers.

As this competition intensifies there may be powerful incentives for regional providers of health care (hospitals, nursing homes, public agencies, etc.) to organize consortia to develop captive registries which compete in wages, benefits, and flexibility of work assignment with freestanding agencies. The obvious incentive of recapturing overhead lost to profit-oriented private sector firms should provide a major financial impetus to such developments.

STRATEGIES FOR COPING WITH SCARCITY

Conventional free-market economists would offer competitors in the increasingly tight nursing market a simple prescription for the problem: raise salaries (particularly in proportion to seniority) until the rate of labor-force participation is adequate to meet nurse staffing needs. This is certainly a strategy which can be pursued for those institutions which have the resources. However, the cost implications of regional bidding wars for nursing personnel are potentially staggering, and in some more heavily regulated settings, simply unsustainable.

More to the point, however, higher wages may not solve the root causes of nurse dissatisfaction. It should be clear from the foregoing discussions that the problem is considerably deeper than relatively low wage levels. Low wages were not perceived by nursing dropouts as a principal reason for dissatisfaction with the profession. Such controversial recruitment practices as cash bounties for nurses reflect more institutional desperation than serious marketing strategy and are likely to disappear as marketing expertise in nurse recruitment grows.

The problem has become serious enough to have spawned a new hospital administrative specialty: nurse recruitment. The competitive market for these specialists is almost as intense as for nurses themselves. Nurse recruiters have professional networks of colleagues who have solved some of the problems of access to steady flows of potential recruits, as well as access to a growing data base about wage and benefits packages, scheduling systems, advertising and recruiting practices, and other key information needed for a hospital to become more competitive. For smaller institutions which may be isolated from pools of potential recruits, a cooperative or consortium approach to nursing recruitment may permit institutions to retain recruitment expertise and spread the cost.[26]

But a marketing perspective on the nursing problem would suggest a deeper analysis of the professional objectives of nurses and of how the work environment can deliver career satisfactions. With average annual turnover rates exceeding 30 percent, nurse retention is a more productive long-term strategy than recruitment.

Focusing on retention will compel hospital administrators and other employers to confront the major sources of job dissatisfaction among nurses. To the extent that nurses continue to be a scarce institutional resource, hospitals, nursing homes, and other institutional providers should develop strategies to maximize the amount of nursing time spent on activities which *only* nurses can perform. There are substantial (but largely hidden) benefits from efficient operation of the service functions in the hospital. Malfunctioning systems for patient transportation, drug distribution, medical records, materials handling, sterile supply, and ancillary services all waste nursing time on the floor and subtract nursing resources from direct patient care, in turn creating job dissatisfaction. The amount of nursing effort tied up in making these systems function for the patient (not to mention the turnover which results) has not been directly estimated, but must be substantial. To the extent that these efforts involve substituting plentiful unskilled, relatively low-pay service workers for scarce nursing personnel, the hospital benefits both financially and in terms of the quality of patient care. The most effective marketing strategy for nurse *retention* may be "simply" the efficient management of administrative and support systems in the hospital.

Complex nurse scheduling systems have been developed which allocate nursing positions flexibly according to the actual nurse acuity (e.g., the amount and type of nursing care), which particular patients require in each nursing unit.[27] These intensity/acuity-based systems can identify precisely areas where nursing resources are stretched too thin and need augmentation, as well as areas where nursing positions are *more* than sufficient for specific patient care needs (offering potential for reassignment). Substantial savings of nursing salary and positions can be achieved by such systems. However, many nurses complain that the system is dehumanizing and creates a larger than desirable pool of floaters, interfering with continuity of both patient care and communication with specific physicians.[28]

Many hospitals have begun to address the flat salary curve/no advancement problem by imaginative efforts to design career ladders. These systems require an investment in performance evaluation and assessment and a willingness to breach seniority if necessary to reward leadership or demonstrated clinical ability. They also require an analysis of job descriptions and systematic examination of the personnel structure in nursing and a willingness to tolerate differential wage increases over a period of time to create effective incentives to retain nurses for longer periods of time.

Many hospitals are beginning to confront the feelings of alienation by involving nurses in designing their work schedules. To the extent that nurses feel they have participated in the process they may be more understanding of the system's failure to allocate them to preferred shifts or duties than if work assignments are perceived to be made arbitrarily.[29] It is highly doubtful that such an approach could be reconciled with intensity-based staffing systems such as those discussed above, but it may be adaptable to a broader range of health care facilities than merely hospitals. Nurse employers will become increasingly sensitive to the variability of full-time versus part-time nurse work habits. Shift differentials in wages have become nearly universal, reflecting the increased difficulties of staffing nights and weekends.

Reexamination of the competiveness of wage and benefits packages will also be helpful. Hospitals competing in the same nursing markets may be offering substantially different inducements to work for them. In this area, nurses will find providers increasingly sensitive to their needs. The movement to provide on-site day care reflects the growing realization of how important a constraint child care may be in the reentry of nurses into part-time or full-time employment. Some hospitals have the financial resources to finance nursing education to the bachelor level by providing tuition aid. In some cases, this represents a reallocation of nursing education resources from diploma programs for which the hospital was directly responsible to financial aid where study is financed in neighboring universities.

Hospitals and other health care providers may discover that one or a number of these strategies will be sufficient to improve retention of experienced nurses to the point where recruitment pressures ease somewhat. Unlike recruitment, which is unquestionably very expensive, many of the retention strategies hinge as much on a changing management philosophy and a changing role for the nurse in the hospital. It is inevitable that facilities and providers will compete through salary and benefits inducements to attract scarce nursing personnel. But those providers who are best able to create a work environment which rewards personal achievement and professional growth and which permits the maximum amount of nursing time to be devoted to the patient care mission that drew nurses into the profession in the first place, will be the most likely winners in the increasingly tight nursing market.

It may be that the nursing profession is one of the casualties of the women's movement in the United States. By devaluing traditionally feminine work roles, feminism may have lowered the occupational status and prestige of nursing as a career for today's young women. Perhaps as the health care system adjusts financially and managerially to the nursing shortage and nursing becomes increasingly attractive financially, men will begin entering the profession in increasing numbers. There is no reason in principle or practice why nursing should be an exclusively feminine occupation. The legitimation of male participation in the profession could help alleviate some of the impending supply problems. Hospitals and other health providers must look to nursing leadership to provide the impetus for this development.

NOTES

1. Joann S. Lublin, "Severe Nurse Shortage Forces Some Hospitals to Close Beds or Units," *The Wall Street Journal,* July 18, 1980, p. 12.
2. Maryann F. Fralic, R.N., "Nursing Shortage: Coping Today and Planning for Tomorrow," *Hospitals,* May 1, 1980, p. 65.
3. Beatrice Kaslisch and Philip Kaslisch, "Nursing Shortage?—Yes," *American Journal of Nursing,* March 1979, p. 469.
4. "R.N. Hospital Vacancy Survey," National Association of Nurses, January 1980.
5. "The Shortage," *RN Magazine,* June 1980, p. 21.
6. "The Nursing Shortage in Illinois Hospitals," Illinois Hospital Association, September 1980, p. 2.

7. Evelyn Moses and Aleda Roth, "Nursepower," *American Journal of Nursing,* October 1979, p. 1745.

8. "Nurse Career Pattern Study," National League of Nursing, Division of Nursing, March 1979, p. 3.

9. Ibid., p. 1.

10. Moses and Roth, "Nursepower," p. 1745.

11. "NLN Notes Decrease in RN Graduates," *American Journal of Nursing,* August 1980, p. 1410.

12. Kaslisch and Kaslisch, "Nursing Shortage?—Yes," p. 471.

13. Fralic, "Nursing Shortage," p. 65.

14. "Nurse Career Pattern Study," p. 3.

15. Tita Corpuz, "Primary Nursing Meets Needs, Expectations of Patients and Staff," *Hospitals,* June 1, 1977, p. 95 ff.

16. Gary Calhoun, "Hospitals are High Stress Employers," *Hospitals,* June 16, 1980, p. 171.

17. Gail Ghigna Hallas, R.N., "Why Nurses are Giving it UP," *RN Magazine,* April 1980, p. 22.

18. Lynn Donovan, "What Nurses Want (And What They're Getting)," *RN Magazine,* April 1980, p. 22.

19. Ibid., p. 27.

20. Lynn Donovan, "What Increases Income Most," *RN Magazine,* February 1980, p. 24.

21. Joyce Alt, Mary Bates, Mary Ann Gilmore, Gary Houston, and Robbie Stone, "Clinical Promotions," *RN Magazine,* June 1980, p. 49.

22. Donovan, "What Nurses Want," p. 27.

23. Tedd Langford and Patricia A. Prescott, "Hospitals and Supplemental Nursing Agencies: An Uneasy Balance," *Journal of Nursing Administration,* November 1979, p. 16 ff.

24. "The Nursing Shortage in Illinois Hospitals," Illinois Hospital Association, p. 7.

25. Ibid.

26. Marvin F. Neely Jr., "Cooperative Recruitment: One Approach," *Hospitals,* July 1, 1980, p. 70.

27. Alt, et al., "Clinical Promotions," p. 49.

28. Diane Meyer, "GRASP—Making the Most of Nursing Budgets," *Hospital Financial Management,* April 1980, p. 32 ff.

29. Fran Cooperrider, "Staff Input in Scheduling Boosts Morale," *Hospitals,* August 1, 1980, p. 59.

10

Conclusion

As the nation struggles to regain control of its economic destiny, resources devoted to paying for health care will inevitably tighten. Public policymakers have worked unsuccessfully for the last 15 years to restrain the growth in health care spending. They appear to be turning away from increased regulation toward the encouragement of constructive economic competition as an approach to restraining costs.

It should be clear to the reader that economic competition in health care is already here—a product of growing numbers of practitioners and a proliferation of new forms of delivering health care as well as of a tightening of the general economy of which health care is only a part. Competition may already have succeeded in capping the demand for hospital services where regulation has failed. The task of policymakers is to capitalize on market trends which are already apparent and to encourage a more efficient use of the purchasing power of the health insurance dollar.

In the first half of this book, an effort was made to analyze the health care market and to explore the competitive forces at work in our health care system. Despite the perennial complaints, hospitals have fared very well in the post-World War II health economy. Increasing prosperity and expanding reimbursement have given rise to the finest network of hospital facilities in the world. Hospitals remain the core of the nation's health care system and demand for hospital services will continue.

However, the cost of hospital care has risen to the point that it has become a political as well as an economic issue. The prudent buyer of health care has begun to seek cost-effective alternatives to hospital care where possible. The analysis above has suggested that those alternatives are both economically attractive and, in some cases, more convenient to the patient than hospital care. The same set of alternatives appear to be available relative to some other types of institutional health care, such as skilled nursing care.

Consumers and insurers appear to be seeking out and demanding these alternatives, as evidenced by the rates of growth in three sectors of the health care market: ambulatory care, aftercare, and health maintenance. In contrast to the growth in these sectors, the demand for inpatient hospital services appears to have leveled off. Per capita consumption of inpatient care actually declined during the last five years. Aggressive attempts to compel economic tradeoffs within the health care market will shrink the demand for inpatient hospital care under a competitive system, threatening established institutions.

As part of this process, the safety net of cost reimbursement will eventually be unravelled. When it is gone, hospitals will no longer be reimbursed for their reasonable cost of providing care. Rather, they will be reimbursed according to what they can get—what the market will bear. Responding to these pressures will place unprecedented stress on management systems and administrative-professional relationships in the hospital.

Facing mounting competitive pressures in their own marketplace, physicians will respond by asserting their economic power. They will develop methods of capturing more of the economic resources associated with their practices through new forms of corporate organization and health delivery. They will share less of these resources with the hospital. Since the physicians are relatively free of regulation and more mobile than the hospital, they can respond more quickly to changing market conditions.

Acting in their own economic interests, physicians can strip away profitable surgical and ancillary services activity and revenue from the hospital. Unless cooperative relations can be forged between the physician and the hospital, the hospital manager will be left with a bundle of services which probably cannot be made economically viable in a highly competitive market. As if this were not enough, constricting capital markets and accelerating inflation will further complicate efforts to preserve the hospital's capital base and operations.

The second half of this book argued that to survive in this market, hospitals will have to change the definition of their business as well as their structure and management philosophy. Those hospitals which cling to the concept of providing inpatient hospital care and traditional hospital-based outpatient care in a single corporation, freestanding organizational framework, will probably not survive in highly competitive markets. Hospitals will be compelled to diversify their offerings of service, softening the mix of services as well as working through cooperative relationships with their medical staffs and other institutions to reach new markets.

In facing these imperatives, hospitals can learn from earlier struggles of many of the nation's largest corporations (which are facing economic pressures fully as serious at a different stage of their evolution) about how to adapt to market change. Hospitals and other health care providers can organize into modern corporations, which introduce managerial and financial controls and economies of scale into a traditionally fragmented marketplace. They can integrate vertically to assure control, managerial or collegial, over less expensive settings for rendering care. They can diversify into related health care services. They can develop flexible new corporate structures to permit them to move to capitalize on new opportunities.

As important as these redefinitions are, the need for re-thinking the troubled compact with the professionals who practice in the hospital is even greater. There is no reason why the modern health care enterprise cannot be managed humanely and why it cannot provide the framework for a satisfying professional practice. Health care managers must insist upon the maintenance of human values in the operation of their facilities. To do this in the face of accelerating economic pressures will be no mean feat. To fail to do it will compromise the quality of patient care and waste precious human resources.

Nurses who feel that they are exploited by the hospital or other providers will continue to leave the profession. Physicians who feel the hospital does not respect their autonomy and professionalism will eventually find a way to practice more medicine without the hospital. Because they deal in human life and death, hospitals will always be stressful places. There are strong incentives for health care managers and professionals to work together cooperatively to minimize the stress.

While it is difficult to find those unwilling to support competition as a concept, few health care providers fully understand that increased economic competition in this market will require unprecedented change in what has traditionally been a conservative, risk-averse industry. Some actors in the system have already recognized that increased competition will require managing for change—creating organizations which are flexible and responsive to the consumer, the professional, and the cost-conscious insurer. Those managers and physicians who shrink, for whatever reasons, from the challenges of constructive entrepreneurship, who are unwilling to alter the way they manage and practice to meet the changing needs of the patient, will eventually be forced out of the health care market.

Appendix

What you need to know about your hospital's competitive position

Market research in the health care field is still in a primitive stage of its evolution. Terminology such as *marketing audit* implies that marketers have developed a precise methodology for determining a hospital's strengths and weaknesses in its markets. This implication is manifestly false. Assessing the hospital's competitive position, while a data-based process, is fully as much an art as a science. While this book has been devoted to attempting to understand the market itself and how it is changing, the purpose of this section is to enable interested hospital administrators, physicians, or others to determine where they stand competitively. This understanding should *precede* constructive action.

If properly conducted, an assessment of your hospital's competitors position is often a humbling experience. The purpose of gathering such information is to show the institution as objectively as possible how it is perceived and used by important external and internal constituencies, relative to competitors. It is sobering to see one's institution as others see it.

Such assessments may also be an important public relations activity, since it may be the first time the hospital has sought external opinions about the quality of its operations. The willingness to listen is an important message to the community, though one which carries with it an implicit obligation to correct perceived deficiencies.

In order to do this, it is essential to gather certain kinds of data about the hospital, its patients, medical staff, and surrounding community. The essential data fall into the following broad groups:

Healthmanpower/
Physician market data:
    Community demand.
    Medical staff practice patterns.
 # RNs available in community
Patient data:
    Insurance coverage, diagnosis, geographical origin.
    Attitudes toward the hospital and its services.

Community data:
    Socioeconomic and demographic characteristics.
    Opinions and attitudes.

Competitor Data:
    Service areas.
    Clinical services—type and volume.
    Feeder systems.

Each of these types of data is discussed below. To the extent that it is impossible to gather this information from published sources or planning agencies, or through formal survey research, much of this information should be available to the perceptive analyst through interviews, dialogue, and anecdotal sources. Shortages of resources for consultants or in-house planning staff do not mean that administrators cannot gather much of this information through other means.

PHYSICIAN MARKET DATA

Hospital marketing specialists often begin their assessments at the level of the hospital and hospital programs. This is a shortsighted approach because, conceptually, hospital utilization is only a subset of the total physician activity in a community. Thus to understand adequately the demand for hospital services in the community one must analyze the organization of the physician marketplace. If a community's physicians are underemployed, that may have a bearing both on their pattern of hospital use and on hospital strategy relative to them.

Hospitals should determine how many physicians practice in the community the hospital services by specialty and, if possible, by nationality (U.S.-trained versus foreign-trained). The office locations (not residences) of these physicians can be plotted on a map, with special designation for those physicians who are members of the hospital's medical staff. This information can be gathered from local medical society directories, or by cross-matching state licensure information against telephone directory listings.

A hospital's patient origins will generally be an amalgamation of the patient origins of the hospital's medical staff's office practices plus the origins of patients who come to the hospital without physician direction (e.g., use of the emergency room). By examining where patients' physicians practice (and in some cases where they live, since they may be treating neighbors and friends), one can often predict with great accuracy the shape of the hospital's so-called primary service area—the area from which the majority of the institution's patients are drawn. The same is true of one's competitors, who may have conveniently published their physicians' office locations in their medical staff directory.

When matched against the socioeconomic and demographic data described below, data on the distribution of your own medical staff's office practices help illuminate how effectively your primary feeder system—physician practices—blanket desirable areas. It can also provide valuable clues to areas which are underserved, in turn guiding physician recruitment and practice location decisions. In addition it can provide a basis for making decisions about where to locate a satellite facility in such a way that practices of your own physicians are minimally disrupted. It is useful to be able to demonstrate this in advance to concerned physicians.

Data on nationality of physicians may be an important variable since many hospital administrators believe that patients prefer to be treated by American-trained physicians if possible. Much physician recruitment strategy in underserved areas focuses on increasing the American-trained complement of physicians on the medical staff. Though surveys at the University of Chicago Medical Center found no differences in patient satisfaction with physicians who are foreign-trained, compared to those trained in the United States, community areas which are served by foreign-trained physicians may be "soft" in terms of possible demand for physician care by American-trained specialists. If obtainable, the percentage of American-trained physicians on competing hospital medical staffs may be an important index of the relative effectiveness of their recruitment efforts.

Determining demand for physician services

One of the findings of the Graduate Medical Education National Advisory Committee (GMENAC) was that there is no accepted scientific method for determining the demand of particular communities for medical generalists and specialists. There are two chief reasons for this. The first is that no one has been able to adequately define what a medical service area is—a geographic unit within which physician use patterns can be captured.* Health planners have struggled unsuccessfully with this problem for many years.

Each possible unit of analysis has some defect. Zipcodes, for example, are used extensively by hospital planners because they are so convenient. They are not always homogeneous in regards to community characteristics however. This is a particular problem in urban areas. For example, the zipcode area surrounding the University of Chicago contains a very prosperous area populated by academics and professionals, a racially mixed middle-class neighborhood, and a rebuilding ghetto neighborhood.

Census tracts are more likely to be homogenous, but are also too small for most analysis and are unlikely to be meaningful in predicting where people get their medical care. City

---

* It may be that health care use patterns vary so drastically from urban to rural and suburban settings that no one methodology can adequately encompass the differences.

boundaries may conceal urban-suburban referral patterns and may not adequately recognize the importation or exportation of medical care from city to suburb or vice versa. Metropolitan areas may be too large an area for assessing demand for all but the most highly specialized medical services. Zipcodes come closest to being most useful but they will be misleading unless some effort is made to superimpose over them what is known about the communities they encompass, such as racial boundaries, and religious or ethnic differences within zipcodes.

The second major reason why it is difficult to determine accurately local physician resource requirements is that consumption of physicians services varies according to the age structure and health status of the population. Thus, physician-to-population ratios for particular medical specialties which apply nationally may not apply to local communities because they may vary in the incidence of the particular illnesses they treat. For these reasons, analysts have been unwilling to apply physician-to-population norms for particular specialties to local communities.

Nevertheless, because it is an imperfect world and management is necessarily imperfect, some guide is better than no guide at all. Figure A–1 below lists GMENAC estimates of national physician manpower requirements for 1990 for most medical specialties expressed in terms of required population per physician. In addition, the figure lists alternative population requirements developed by the specialty societies themselves or by other groups. These estimates should be modified intuitively by what is known about the health status and age structure of the community relative to national norms. They are more likely to be useful guides to planning in small cities and suburban areas than in large inner city or completely rural areas. In these latter communities, people may be more willing to travel greater distances (e.g., to tertiary centers) to receive certain types of quality care.

Travel time is an important intervening variable in assessing demand. Research at the University of Chicago Medical Center has suggested that Chicago suburban populations are generally located an average of about 15 minutes from their family doctor, while inner city populations may travel one-half hour or more to reach their physicians. Acceptable travel

FIGURE A-1
Estimates of population required per health professional

| Specialty | GMENAC (1990) | GAO report | | HEW review of manpower requirements standards |
		Specialty board	Specialty society	
General family practice	4,000		2,500	2,000–4,000 [PJ]*
General pediatrics	8,100		2000–2500	10,000 [PJ]
Pediatric allergy	270,570			
Pediatric cardiology	211,750			
Pediatric endocrinology	304,390			
Pediatric hematology/oncology	147,600			
Pediatric nephrology	695,750			
Neonatology	187,320			
General internal medicine	3,500			3,846; 5,000; 20,000 [PJ]
Allergy/immunology	118,800			25,000 [PJ]
Cardiology	31,420			25,000; 77,000 [PJ]
Endocrinology	118,800			
Gastroenterology	37,460		50,000	50,000 [PJ]
Hematology/oncology	27,060			
Infectious disease	108,230			
Nephrology	88,550			
Pulmonary disease	67,640			100,000 [PJ]
Rheumatology	143,240			

Neurology	44,275			
Dermatology	35,040	31,250		40,000; 50,000 (PJ)
Psychiatry (general)	6,325	25,000		4,000–143,000 (PJ)
Child psychiatry	27,060			
Obstetrics/gynecology	10,150	10,000		22,560; 10,000–11,000 (Need) (PJ)
General surgery	10,360			9,000–10,000; 11,650 (PJ) (Demand)
Neurosurgery	91,890			77,000–125,000; 161,930 (PJ) (Demand)
Ophthalmology	20,990			20,000 (PJ)
Orthopedic surgery	16,130			20,000–35,000 (PJ); 28,900 (Demand)
Otolaryngology	30,440		28,600–40,000	25,000–33,000; (PJ) 70,400 (Demand)
Plastic surgery	90,190		50,000	50,000–150,000 (PJ)
Thoracic surgery	118,800	100,000	100,000	50,000–150,000 (PJ)
Urology	31,625	25,000–60,000 35,000–40,000	30,000	21,300–50,000; 55,227 (PJ) (Demand)
Emergency medicine	18,040			

* PJ = professional judgement—the opinion of health professionals or health manpower experts.

Sources: GMENAC: *Report of the Graduate Medical Education National Advisory Committee to the Secretary, Department of Health and Human Services*, United States Department of Health and Human Services Public Health Service, Health Research Administration Volume 1, September 1980.

United States Comptroller General, *Report to the Congress of the United States: Are Enough Physicians of the Right Types Trained in the United States?* United States General Accounting Office, May 16, 1978.

United States Department of Health Education and Welfare, *Review of Health Manpower Population Requirements Standards*, Public Health Service, Health Research Administration, October 1976.

Reports from specialty societies including: American Urological Association.

time for given populations is difficult to assess without directly surveying them, but it has an important role in determining whether a community is over or underserved. If patients must travel more than 20 minutes to reach their family doctor it is reasonable to assume that their area may need more primary physicians.

As mentioned in the chapter on the physician and the hospital, physician market data is essential for physician recruitment and development. It can help members of a group practice determine the competitive implications of adding new physicians to their group by identifying specialty gaps in particular community areas. It can also help in decisions concerning possible branches in newly developing areas. While it is necessary to make some assumptions about how far people are willing to travel to receive physician care, the data can also be useful in identifying which groups of physicians are likely to be economically affected by new hospital satellite services or by joint ventures between the hospital and medical staff.

Physician practice patterns

However, data on geographical location of outlets for physician care is not enough. Hospital administrators must have a detailed knowledge of the practice patterns of their medical staff. Most administrators know, either intuitively or from some form of continuing monitoring, who the key admitters to the hospital are. However, intuition is no substitute for facts. Although key continuing activity data should be gathered by admitting and billing reports, additional information should be gathered by the most appropriate means. The essential practice data should include: total annual office visit volume, total annual hospital admissions to all hospitals at which the physician practices, and the share of those admissions which occur at the particular hospital as well as the factors which govern that share. If the patient practices in a referral specialty, it is important to know the proportions of his or her visits and admissions which are generated by medical staff colleagues and the proportion generated by outside physicians. The physician's age and mode of practice (solo, partnership, and group) should also be known.

For surgical specialties the volume of procedures performed and the share performed at each of the hospitals
at which the surgeon has privileges should be ascertained.
Here supporting relationships with anaesthesiologists, radiologists, and pathologists are particularly crucial in determining the hospital's share of the surgeon's utilization as
well as the relative accessibility of operating room time.

In addition to these data it is important to know which
ancillary services the physician depends upon and how reliable he or she finds the service in hospital based departments.
This information may be useful in uncovering important peer
ties within the institution which can form the basis for alli-
ances or blocs of physicians. In addition, the colleagues who
generate inhouse consultations for the physician as well as
those relied upon for consultation should be uncovered. If
these supportive relationships are not satisfactory in one
hospital, they may be grounds for moving marginal activity
to other institutions.

The goal of gathering this information is to determine what
share of the total hospital activities of the medical staff one's
particular hospital commands. Gathered over a period of
time, these data will provide critical information as to
whether one is gaining or losing "market share" of particular
physicians' admissions. The information on support departments and relationships of dependence with other medical
staff may provide clues as to why the share of a particular
physician's utilization is increasing or decreasing.

The market share information on particular physicians
is also an important way of identifying key competing hospitals for particular clinical services. While it is important to
know who your key admitters are, it is also important to
know how many of your medical staff are using the hospital
as a primary hospital and how many as a back-up facility.
This may be the best way of learning what types of hospital
and medical staff support may be necessary to encourage
the physician to use the hospital as a primary rather than
back-up facility.

Physician data is vitally important to a comprehensive
marketing audit. If no other data were gathered, this data

is essential to effective strategic management of the hospital. There is no substitute for a detailed knowledge of the physician marketplace and the share of physician activity the hospital commands. This data will provide clues to how much marginal utilization can be created through internal discussion and negotiation with existing medical staff before moving into more risky, costly new program development.

Hospitals with utilization problems frequently look beyond their current complement of medical staff to new recruitment and programs before identifying how much of the problem could be solved by serving existing medical staff more effectively. Because this approach commits the administrator to understanding how the hospital can better support physician practice, it is an effective way of legitimating the manager's presence on what some physicians may feel is alien turf. If this data can be gathered under medical staff auspices, through the chief of staff or medical staff president, so much the better.

PATIENT DATA

Nearly all hospitals track gross patient activity, such as inpatient occupancy and outpatient or emergency visits. However, some hospitals do not routinely monitor changes in the characteristics of their patients. Understanding the composition, origins, and attitudes of patients using the hospital is the second task of a marketing audit. A hospital's financial viability may be seriously affected by shifts in patient population or characteristics. For example, most hospitals try to achieve a sufficient mass of patients with relatively generous health insurance benefits so that the hospital can recover its costs and generate sufficient net income to pay for new programs, capital improvements, and equipment. Hospitals with a majority of patients which are publicly funded (medicare and medicaid) are unreasonably exposed to the vicissitudes of state and federal fiscal policy as well as to extraordinary audit vulnerability. Unless a hospital monitors the insurance status (payer mix) of its patients, it may experience a deterioration of its financial position even if its occupancy remains high. While it is often impossible to obtain, information on other hospitals' mix of payer can help assess the strength of their financial position, and consequently, the extent of the pressure on them to reach out to new patients.

If government moves toward possible purchase of services on a diagnosis rather than on a per diem basis, it will become increasingly important for the hospital to understand and monitor changes in the diagnostic mix in the hospital—the mixture of medical problems the hospital treats. This mix will have a hidden but potentially significant effect on the hospital's costs, since sicker patients consume larger portions of the hospital's resources, which insurance systems may or may not reimburse fully.

Most administrators obtain some understanding of the geographical origins of patients by conducting periodic or ongoing patient origin studies. Since communities are undergoing constant change it is important to know where one's patients are coming from, by clinical services (medicine, surgery, pediatrics, etc.) if possible. When matched with socio-economic data on the community, patient origin data can help explain which services may be contributing more or less than their share of net hospital revenues. When matched to diagnostic data, patient origin data can help identify areas from which patients with particular conditions, or requiring certain sophisticated medical procedures (CAT scans, cardiac catheterization, etc.) are drawn.

However, the most important use of patient origin information is in identifying competitors. While individual hospitals can gather data and analyze changes in patient origins within their own institutions, only data gathered from all providers in a given area will help determine a hospital's market share for particular areas. Overlap between hospital primary service areas (technically defined as the zipcodes which, when added cumulatively, account for 70 percent or more of the hospital's inpatient admissions), indicates which hospitals are pulling patients from the same area. While this overlap may mirror sharing of medical staff (e.g., medical staff with privileges in more than one institution), it may also be attributed to unique programs offered at one or another institution. Knowledge of one's competitors is the beginning of a competitive strategy. Assessment of the competition will be discussed below.

Patient satisfaction

Many hospitals have conducted patient satisfaction surveys to help identify aspects of the hospital's programs that are drawing cards and those which, all other factors being equal, discourage further patronage. While it is true that the physician controls where his or her patient is hospitalized, failure to render compassionate, efficient hospital care may cause the patient to request or demand that the physician hospitalize the patient at another institution for a subsequent medical problem.

An effective patient satisfaction study provides the patient an opportunity to react to every major aspect of his or her encounter with the hospital from admission to discharge. It should probe the responsiveness and courtesy of all staff groups who have contact with the patient, including physicians and nursing personnel. It should also contain sufficient background information on the patient (clinical service, age, sex, payer, race, referral status, etc.), to enable the analyst to identify those groups which may be more or less satisfied with hospital care.

These studies can be useful as ongoing activities to monitor changes in the hospital's ambience and serve as a guide to the need for management or personnel changes. They are an important device for holding hospital managers accountable for the high quality of personal service rendered the patient. As Peter Drucker suggested, marketing must permeate every aspect of the institution's transaction with the "customer." Those individuals who render hands-on service to the patient must understand that their courtesy and efficiency may have a bearing on the long-term viability of the hospital, and they must be held accountable for behavior which may affect the hospital's service to patients.

As a guide to how well the hospital is doing in the aggregate, however, patient origin studies can be very misleading. Most patient satisfaction surveys produce very high rates of overall satisfaction with hospital care. Survey researchers refer to this phenomenon as "positive response bias." Because people are somewhat intimidated by hospitals generally and may be concerned about the impact of negative comments on their own physicians or nursing personnel, patient satisfaction survey results frequently reflect near unanimous approval. Another reason for this may be that dissatisfied patients have voted with their feet and asked their physician to hospitalize them elsewhere. Thus, the population evaluating the hospital may have been self-selected from a larger universe which may be less favorably disposed to the institution.

For whatever reason, the high positive response bias should stimulate caution before trumpeting absolute values (e.g., "96 percent of our patients loved our service"). Rather, attention should focus on areas which attracted a disproportionate amount of criticism. By examining areas or personnel who produced significantly lower rates of overall satisfaction, hospital administration and medical staff can identify areas of weakness. Thus analysis of patient satisfaction frequently turns on identifying "outliers" and in attempting to identify those groups of patients which are disproportionately unhappy with the hospital's services. A hospital which learns that 85 percent of its patients are satisfied with overall care, but also learns that only 45 percent of its charge-paying patients and 55 percent of its younger patients are satisfied, should be disturbed by what it has learned.

While it is obviously important to make use of patient satisfaction data to improve the hospital's service to the patient, the hospital administrator should remember that the majority of patient use of the facility is generated by the physician. Efforts to market directly to patients which bypass the physician may threaten the medical staff and bring counterproductive results. While a marketing-oriented hospital must be responsive to changing patient needs and perceptions, it must remember that the *physician* is the core market of the hospital. Satisfying the patient is a necessary, but not sufficient, condition of generating further business.

COMMUNITY DATA

Since the premise of this book is that hospitals must change their programs and structures to accommodate changing social needs, attention must be focused on how the community's social and economic composition is changing and on its perceived health care needs.

Demographic and socioeconomic data

With the publication of data from the 1980 census, hospitals will have no excuse for not understanding the changes taking place in their communities. The census will not only help managers assess whether adequate populations exist in the community for certain medical and related services but also help them understand such factors as population growth, changes in age and family structure, income trends, and other vital information about the patients currently or potentially served by hospital programs.

Changing patterns of family income, for example, may help administrators predict changes in the insurance status of their patients and anticipated bad debt and free care performance. Family income data will also help assess physician income opportunities in the community. These data can in turn lead to decisions about how to structure the hospital to render ambulatory and other services. If there have been sharp increases in elderly population hospitals may have added impetus to diversify into aftercare services to meet their needs. Changes in the proportion of children or women of childbearing age may help establish future demand for age and sex-specific clinical services such as pediatrics and obstetrics and gynecology.

Population growth from 1970 to 1980 will provide planners and decision-makers with key information on how and where to diversify the hospital's feeder system. Identification of areas of rapid population growth will help in locating satellite facilities or to justify programmatic changes, such as adding beds or operating suites. In rapidly expanding areas, population growth estimates have led planning agencies to increase the number of beds or clinical services in their regions. The sooner hospitals have a grasp of where underserved populations exist, the more quickly they can respond to meet their needs.

Consumer attitudes

Finally, by conducting surveys of health care consumers in the community, hospitals can identify perceived programmatic strengths and weaknesses of their own as well as of competing institutions. Here it is important to gather data which illuminates different traits or features of the hospital and its competitors (strength of the medical staff, quality of nursing, ambience, "prestige," image of the patient population served by the hospital, etc.). The extent of past use of the hospital, and the degree to which the image of the facility is conditioned by direct use or by "reputation," should also be determined. Since not all patients have a regular physician or source of care, knowing who these patients are can be important in identifying potential markets which are *not* mediated directly by physicians for promotion of the hospital's services. Finally, survey instruments should contain sufficient personal detail (age, sex, marital status, family size, race, income, occupation, etc.) so that profiles of respondents having relatively positive or negative perceptions of the hospital relative to competitors can be constructed statistically.

Community opinion data can also be important in identifying particular image problems in the hospital. For example, a hospital's emergency room may be a disproportionate contributor to the hospital's community image because of the high level of self-referral and the 24-hour-a-day nature of the program. If a hospital's emergency room has the reputation of rendering impersonal care, or of having excessive waiting time, the negative community image may reflect on the rest of the hospital's programs.

Just as patient satisfaction studies have a positive public relations impact by letting patients know that their opinions are important to hospital management, community surveys may have a similar impact on community opinion about the hospital. A more direct method of gathering the same information at much lower cost may be to assemble small face-to-face groups of community opinion leaders, or individuals drawn from specific community areas, to discuss health services and the role of the hospital in them. Called "focus groups," these guided discussions begin with broad issues and opinions about health facilities and services and narrow gradually to the particular institution and competitors in question.

Corporations use focus groups to develop product concepts and promotional ideas and to pre-test advertising copy and survey instruments to measure audience response to advertising campaigns. Frequently, community groups will agree to sponsor such discussions to permit a more objective framework for the discussion. Leading such groups is something of an art, and consultants are frequently a good investment. For hospitals or other organizations contemplating major surveys, focus groups are a low-cost pre-testing procedure which can significantly improve questionnaire design.

COMPETITOR DATA BASE

In an increasingly competitive market it is essential to understand the products, strengths, and weaknesses of competing institutions. These institutions include not only neighboring hospitals but also so-called single service providers such as ambulatory sugical centers and urgent care centers. Several critical pieces of information on competitors will already have been gathered in the three data groups discussed above.

First, the share of hospitalization which your medical staff may be generating for competing institutions is vital information. Having identified key competitors for existing business of current medical staff, it is important to identify as well the reasons why medical staff are splitting their admissions. It may be possible to identify areas where competing administrators are not responding to physician needs, pinpointing areas where your organization may be able to move to satisfy these needs. Intelligence about medical staff moral and political movements may be important in identifying physicians who are under pressure or who are looking for other outlets for care.

A dramatic example of how this information can be used occurred several years ago in Florida. A national hospital management firm acquired a small hospital no more than several hundred yards from a very large and troubled tertiary hospital. Preliminary scouting of the acquired hospital's medical staff revealed major internal divisions at the neighboring hospital, including perceptions among the larger hospital's primary care physicians and cardiologists that their needs were not being met. The firm designed a primary care oriented program for the small hospital and developed support facilities for cardiac catheterization and cardiac surgery, and was able to build their percentage of occupancy into the high 80s within 18 months by pulling utilization away from the larger hospital. The larger hospital's occupancy and financial condition were significantly damaged.

Second, by identifying areas of overlap in hospital primary service areas it is possible to identify competitors in those areas. Since hospitals will try to capture market share in growing areas, time series data is particularly important in analyzing changes in patient origins. Having identified competitors in specific areas, one can develop a profile of services available at competing institutions to attempt to understand the factors which may have led to their growth. Health systems agencies have enormously simplified gathering detailed program information on competing institutions through appropriateness review of key clinical services. Since most of the utilization and cost data gathered through appropriateness review is public information, it is possible to construct a product line profile of clinical services of one's own hospital relative to competitors. This data base will help guide program expansion, and more precisely identify competitors by key clinical program.

In addition to the above information, it is important to identify, by geography and hospital linkage if not in terms of actual utilization, the organized outlets for ambulatory care in the community. These include hospital emergency rooms and organized outpatient clinics, public health clinics, community health centers, freestanding urgent care centers and ambulatory surgical programs, and large multispecialty group practices. While health systems agencies or other planning bodies, or local hospital associations, may gather extensive data on hospital-based or public health care programs, it is virtually impossible to gather information on the volume of services private physicians control. To the extent possible, however, at least the number of physicians practicing in office settings should be determined.

It is often difficult for administrators or physicians to accept the fact that local demand for most forms of health care is relatively finite, and that changes in a hospital's outpatient or inpatient utilization may frequently be explained by program changes of neighboring facilities or by increasing numbers of physician providers. Strategies to affect the hospital's market share and position must inevitably be developed in the context of competing providers, since existing and contemplated program changes by competitors may significantly affect the future market and financial viability of programs the hospital is contemplating.

A marketing approach to developing new health care programs begins with the recognition that the feasibility of program changes rests upon the competitive outlook for those programs. Hospitals have been compelled by Certificate of Need to conduct feasibility studies for new capital programs. But willingness to apply the same types of criteria and methodologies to such matters as the recruitment of new physicians or the development of new clinical programs has lagged in many hospitals. Until boards of trustees begin to apply the same criteria for evaluating new lines of business in their facilities that they do to evaluating potential new business ventures in the corporate world, hospitals may squander precious resources by allocating them without a clear notion of the potential market for the services they are intended to offer.

The development of a comprehensive marketing data base is an essential precondition to making informed strategic choices about a hospital's programs, facilities, and promotional approach. Smaller institutions may have limited resources to engage in extensive survey research. But they can rely on increasingly complete local data bases assembled by their HSAs and on informal, less costly means of gathering data, such as focus groups. Keeping abreast of developments among the practicing physicians in a community, and developing relationships of confidence sufficient to help pinpoint clinical strengths and weaknesses of competing institutions, will become more and more important as the market for hospital services continues to tighten. Those administrators and trustees who are reluctant to gather and capitalize upon such information may be left behind.

FIGURE A–2
Nonfederal physicians, civilian population, physician-population ratios and rank by state, 1978

State	Civilian population (7–1–78)	Nonfederal physicians (12–31–78) Total	Nonfederal physicians (12–31–78) Patient care	Physicians per 100,000 population Total	Physicians per 100,000 population Patient care	Rank of physician-population ratio by state Total	Rank of physician-population ratio by state Patient care
Alabama	3,719,000	4,554	3,833	122	103	45	45
Alaska	379,000	460	378	121	100	46	46
Arizona	2,327,000	4,918	3,732	211	160	11	11
Arkansas	2,176,000	2,610	2,165	120	99	47	47
California	22,021,000	52,194	41,296	237	188	6	6
Colorado	2,626,000	5,600	4,548	213	173	10	7
Connecticut	3,084,000	7,705	6,054	250	196	5	4
Delaware	577,000	972	805	168	140	22	20
D.C.	666,000	3,491	2,576	524	387	1	1
Florida	8,499,000	18,353	13,584	216	160	8	12
Georgia	5,024,000	7,259	6,090	144	121	35	34
Hawaii	838,000	1,808	1,447	216	173	9	10
Idaho	872,000	1,010	847	116	97	48	48
Illinois	11,205,000	20,628	16,602	184	148	18	17
Indiana	5,368,000	6,993	5,807	130	108	41	43
Iowa	2,895,000	3,635	3,035	126	105	44	44
Kansas	2,323,000	3,618	2,938	156	126	29	30
Kentucky	3,464,000	4,699	3,873	136	112	39	39
Louisiana	3,934,000	5,955	4,833	151	123	33	32
Maine	1,081,000	1,752	1,378	162	127	23	27
Maryland	4,100,000	10,390	7,808	253	190	4	5
Massachusetts	5,761,000	14,985	11,517	260	200	3	3
Michigan	9,178,000	14,290	11,688	156	127	30	28
Minnesota	4,006,000	7,676	6,369	192	159	13	13
Mississippi	2,383,000	2,571	2,179	108	91	50	50
Missouri	4,840,000	7,839	6,150	162	127	24	29
Montana	779,000	1,024	878	131	113	40	38
Nebraska	1,553,000	2,338	1,898	151	122	34	33
Nevada	651,000	925	758	142	116	36	36
New Hampshire	867,000	1,542	1,190	178	137	19	22
New Jersey	7,303,000	13,820	11,029	189	151	14	15
New Mexico	1,196,000	1,869	1,434	156	120	28	35
New York	17,722,000	47,021	36,307	265	205	2	2
North Carolina	5,478,000	8,428	6,777	154	124	32	31
North Dakota	640,000	825	707	129	110	42	41
Ohio	10,736,000	17,325	14,477	161	135	25	23
Oklahoma	2,852,000	3,650	3,120	128	109	43	42
Oregon	2,440,000	4,546	3,615	186	148	17	18
Pennsylvania	11,740,000	22,149	17,883	189	152	15	14
Rhode Island	931,000	1,967	1,609	211	173	12	8
South Carolina	2,852,000	3,873	3,159	136	111	38	40
South Dakota	683,000	723	611	106	89	51	51
Tennessee	4,336,000	6,808	5,614	157	129	26	24
Texas	12,869,000	20,143	16,540	157	129	27	25
Utah	1,302,000	2,225	1,829	171	140	21	19
Vermont	487,000	1,075	841	221	173	7	9
Virginia	4,994,000	8,653	6,958	173	139	20	21
Washington	3,722,000	6,981	5,553	188	149	16	16
West Virginia	1,859,000	2,565	2,123	138	114	37	37
Wisconsin	4,677,000	7,271	5,999	155	128	31	26
Wyoming	420,000	479	394	114	94	49	49

Source: Wunderman, Lorna E. *Physician Distribution and Medical Licensure in the U.S., 1978* (Chicago: Center for Health Research and Development, American Medical Association, 1979).

FIGURE A–3

Ratio percent of projected supply to estimated requirements—1990

	Ratio percent	Require-ments	Surplus (shortage)
Shortages:			
Child psychiatry......................	45%	9,000	(4,900)
Emergency medicine	70%	13,500	(4,250)
Preventive medicine	75%	7,300	(1,750)
General psychiatry	80%	38,500	(8,000)
Near Balance:			
Hematology/oncology—			
internal medicine....................	90%	9,000	(700)
Dermatology	105%	6,950	400
Gastroenterology—			
internal medicine....................	105%	6,500	400
Osteopathic general			
practice............................	105%	22,000	1,150
Family practice.......................	105%	61,300	3,100
General Internal Medicine	105%	70,250	3,550
Otolaryngology.......................	105%	8,000	500
General pediatrics and			
subspecialties	115%	36,400	4,950
Surpluses:			
Urology...............................	120%	7,700	1,650
Orthopedic surgery	135%	15,100	5,000
Ophthalmology	140%	11,800	4,700
Thoracic surgery	140%	2,050	850
Infectious diseases—			
internal medicine	145%	2,250	1,000
Obstetrics/gynecology	145%	24,000	10,450
Plastic surgery	145%	2,700	1,200
Allergy/immunology—			
internal medicine....................	150%	2,050	1,000
General surgery	150%	23,500	11,800
Nephrology—			
internal medicine....................	175%	2,750	2,100
Rheumatology—			
internal medicine....................	175%	1,700	1,300
Cardiology—			
internal medicine....................	190%	7,750	7,150
Endocrinology—			
internal medicine....................	190%	2,050	1,800
Neurosurgery	190%	2,650	2,450
Pulmonary—			
internal medicine....................	195%	3,600	3,350
Estimated:			
Physical medicine and			
rehabilitation	75%	3,200	(800)
Anaesthesiology.......................	95%	21,000	(1,550)
Nuclear medicine.....................	n.a.	4,000	n.a.
Pathology.............................	125%	13,500	3,350
Radiology.............................	155%	18,000	9,800
Neurology	160%	5,500	3,150

Note: The requirements in the six estimated specialties should be considered as rough approximations and tentative. They were estimated crudely after a review of the literature.

n.a. = not available.

Source: Report of the Graduate Medical Education National Advisory Committee to the Secretary, Department of Health and Human Services, September 1980, p. 4.

BIBLIOGRAPHY

"An Acute Shortage of Nurses." *Newsweek,* September 2, 1980, pp. 93–95.

Alt, Joyce M.; Mary D. Bates; Mary Ann Gilmore; Gary R. Houston; and Robbie S. Stoner. "Clinical Promotions." *RN Magazine,* June 1980, pp. 49–51.

Altman, Stuart H. *Present and Future Supply of Registered Nurses.* Washington, D.C.: Department of Health and Human Services, November 1971.

Amado, Anthony. "Cost of Terminal Care: Home Hospice *vs.* Hospital." *Nursing Outlook,* August 1979, pp. 522–26.

American Hospital Association. *Advertising by Hospitals—Guidelines.* Chicago: American Hospital Association, 1977.

_____. *Hospital Statistics, 1980.* Chicago: American Hospital Association, 1980.

_____. *National Hospital Panel Survey.* Chicago: American Hospital Association, 1980.

American Hospital Association Department of Financial Management Systems, Staff Issue Paper. *Financing Ambulatory Care.* Chicago: American Hospital Association, 1980.

American Medical Association. *Profile of Medical Practice, 1979.* Chicago: American Medical Association Center for Health Services Research and Development, 1979.

American Medical Association Center for Health Services Research and Development. "Research Notes." Chicago: American Medical Association, Spring 1981.

American Medical Association Council on Medical Service. "Health Maintenance Organizations." Chicago: American Medical Association. (Distributed as information for the House of Delegates and contains background data for Council on Medical Service Report A [A–80] *Study of the Health Maintenance Organizations.*)

American Medical Association Report of the Council on Medical Service. *Study of Health Maintenance Organizations.* Report A (A–80).

American Nurses' Association. *Facts About Nursing 76–77.* Kansas City, Mo.: American Nurses Association, 1977.

"ANA Convention Briefs." *Modern Healthcare,* July 1980.

Anderson, Odin. "Why We Are Where We Are." University of Chicago Center for Health Administrations Studies Workshop, January 29, 1981.

Araujo, Marianne. "Creative Nursing Administration Sets Climate for Retention." *Hospitals,* May 1, 1980, p. 72.

Arthur Young and Company. *Home Health: An Industry Composite.* August 1980.

Bailey, R. M. "Economies of Scale and Medical Practice." In *Empirical Studies in Health Economics,* edited by Herber Klarman. Baltimore: Johns Hopkins University Press, 1970.

Bardossi, Karen. "Why BSN Programs Drive Nurses Crazy." *RN Magazine,* February 1980, pp. 53–63.

Barron, Ellen ana James K. Knoble. "Ambulatory Surgery Offers Quality, Savings." *Hospitals,* February 1, 1980, pp. 74–76.

Bays, Carson. "Cost Comparison of For-Profit and Non-Profit Hospitals." *Social Science and Medicine* 13C, December 1979, pp. 219–25.

Berk, Aviva Ancona and Thomas C. Chalmers. "Cost and Efficacy of the Substitution of Ambulatory for Inpatient Care." *New England Journal of Medicine,* February 12, 1981, pp. 393–97.

Biles, Brian; Carl Schramm; and J. Graham Atkinson. "Hospital Cost Inflation Under State Rate-Setting Programs." *New England Journal of Medicine,* September 18, 1980, pp. 664–68.

Boyer, Cheryl. "The Use of Supplemental Nurses: Why, Where and How?" *Journal of Nursing Administration,* March 1979, pp. 56–60.

"A Bright Prognosis for the Once-Frail HMO's." *Business Week,* October 27, 1980, pp. 108–16.

Brown, Montague. "HCMR Interview: Michael D. Bromberg, Esq." *Health Care Management Review,* Fall 1980, pp. 87–95.

_____. "MultiHospital Systems: Trends, Issues, Prospects." Prepared for HRET Invitational Conference on Multihospital Systems, Washington, D.C., March 18, 1980.

_____., and Barbara McCool. *MultiHospital Systems: Strategies for Organization and Management.* Rockville, Md.: Aspen Systems Corporation, 1980.

Calhoun, Gary L. "Hospitals are High-Stress Employers." *Hospitals,* June 16, 1980, pp. 171–76.

Capuzzi, Cecelia. "Power and Interest Groups: A Study of ANA and AMA." *Nursing Outlook,* August 1980, pp. 478–82.

Chandler, Alfred. *Strategy and Structure: Chapters in the History of the American Industrial Enterprise.* Cambridge, Mass.: MIT Press, 1962.

Christianson, Jon B., and Walter McClure. "Competition in the Delivery of Medical Care." *New England Journal of Medicine,* June 7, 1979, pp. 812–18.

"City, County Contracts Lead to Hospital Sales." *Modern Healthcare,* September 1980, p. 44.

Clark, Robert. "Does the Non-Profit Form Fit the Hospital-Industry?" *Harvard Law Review,* August 1980, pp. 1417–89.

Coelen, Craig and Daniel Sullivan. "An Analysis of the Effects of Prospective Reimbursement Programs on Hospital Expenditures." *Health Care Financing Review,* Winter 1981, pp. 1–40.

Collum, Emily W. "Bringing Nurse Education out of Isolation." *Hospitals,* June 16, 1980, pp. 195–98.

"Congress Expected to 'Continue' Nursing Funds." *American Journal of Nursing,* August 1980, pp. 1387–92.

Constantinou, S., and Gordon Hatcher. "The Relationship Between the Supply of Physicians and Surgical Costs." *Dimensions in Health Service,* January 1979, pp. 30–33.

Cooperrider, Fran. "Staff Input in Scheduling Boosts Morale. *Hospitals,* August 1, 1980, pp. 59–61.

Corpuz, Tita. "Primary Nursing Meets Needs, Expectations of Patients and Staff." *Hospitals,* June 1, 1977, pp. 95–100.

Coyne, Joseph S. "Nonprofit Hospital Groups Make a Move on Investor-Owned Systems." *Modern Healthcare,* November 1980, pp. 82–88.

Cunningham, Frances, and John Williamson, M.D. "How Does the Quality of Health Care in HMO's Compare to Those in Other Settings? An Analytic Review of the Literature 1958–1979." *Group Health Journal,* Winter 1980, pp. 2–23.

Curran, J. P. *People Taking Care of People—A Report on the Home Health Care Service Industry—Three New Recommendations.* New York: Woody Gundy Incorporated, September 29, 1980.

Davis, James E., and Don E. Detmer. "The Ambulatory Surgical Unit." *Annals of Surgery,* June 1972.

Demkovich, Linda E. "Choosing Hospitals for the Poor—Should the States Have That Power?" *National Journal,* September 13, 1980, pp. 1516–18.

————. "Hospitals Adopting the Old Axiom—In Numbers There is Strength." *National Journal,* August 9, 1980, pp. 1316–20.

————. "New Congressional Health Leaders—The Emphasis is on Competition." *National Journal,* July 5, 1980, pp. 1093–97.

Derzon, Robert; Lawrence Lewin; and J. Michael Watt. "Not-for-Profit Chains Share in Multi-hospital Boom." *Hospitals,* May 16, 1981, pp. 65–71.

"Dialysis Reimbursement Squeeze Spurs New Management Services." *Modern Healthcare,* August 1980, p. 80.

Dietz, Jean. "Useless Hospitalizations Cited in Report on Nursing Home Beds." *Boston Globe,* May 3, 1979.

DiPaolo, Vince. "Tight Money, Higher Interest Rates Slow Nursing Home Systems Growth." *Modern Healthcare,* June 1980, pp. 76–84.

Dolan, Andrew K. "Antitrust Law and Physician Dominance of Other Health Practitioners." *Journal of Health, Politics, Policy and Law* 4, no. 4 (Winter 1980): 675–89.

Donabedian, Avedis. *Benefits in Medical Care Administration.* Cambridge, Mass.: Harvard University Press, 1976.

Donovan, Lynn. "The Shortage." *RN Magazine,* June 1980, pp. 21–27.

————. "What Increases Income Most." *RN Magazine,* February 1980.

————. "What Nurses Want (And What They're Getting)." *RN Magazine,* April 1980, pp. 22–30.

Drucker, Peter. *The Practice of Management.* New York: Harper & Row, 1954.

Dunlop, Burton. *The Growth of Nursing Home Care.* Lexington, Mass.: Lexington Books, 1979.

Eamer, Richard K. "Why Proprietary Hospitals are More Efficient and Cost Effective." *Modern Healthcare,* April 1978, p. 60.

"Earnings Survey." *Medical Economics,* September 15, 1980, pp. 99–107.

Ellwood, Paul M., and Michael E. Herbert. "Health Care: Should Industry Buy it or Sell it?" *Harvard Business Review,* July–August 1973.

Enthoven, Alain C. "Consumer Centered *vs.* Job Centered Health Insurance." *Harvard Business Review,* January–February 1979, pp. 141–52.

————. *Health Plan: The Only Practical Solution to the Soaring Cost of Medical Care.* Reading, Mass.: Addison-Wesley Publishing, 1980.

Ernst, Richard. "Ancillary Production and the Size of Physicians' Practice." *Inquiry* 13 (December 1976), pp. 371–81.

Evans, Frank O. Jr., M.D. "Physician-Based Group Insurance." *The New England Journal of Medicine,* June 15, 1978, pp. 1280–83.

Federation of American Hospitals. *1979–1980 Directory of Investor Owned Hospitals and Hospital Management Companies.* Little Rock, Ark.: Federation of American Hospitals, 1979.

_____. *1981 Directory of Investor Owned Hospitals and Hospital Management Companies.* Little Rock, Ark.: Federation of American Hospitals, 1980.

"Federal HMO Funds May Run Out." *Modern Healthcare,* February 1981, p. 16.

Fisher, Charles R. "Differences by Age Groups in Health Care Spending." *Health Care Financing Review,* Spring 1980, pp. 65–90.

Ford, Loretta. "Nursing at the Cutting Edge of Health Services Reform." *American Journal of Nursing,* August 1980, pp. 1476–79.

Fralic, Maryann F. "Nursing Shortage: Coping Today and Planning for Tomorrow." *Hospitals,* May 1, 1980, pp. 65–67.

Freshnock, Larry J., and Lynn E. Jensen. "The Changing Structure of Medical Group Practice, 1969 to 1980." *Journal of the American Medical Association,* June 5, 1981, pp. 2173–76.

Fries, James F. "Aging, Natural Death, and the Compression of Morbidity." *New England Journal of Medicine,* July 17, 1980, pp. 130–35.

Gabel, Jon R., and Michael Redisch. "Alternative Physician Payment Methods: Incentives, Efficiency, and National Health Insurance." *Milbank Memorial Fund Quarterly/Health and Society* 57, no. 1 (1979):38–59.

Geisel, Jerry. "25% of HMOs Could Die of Thirst if Congress Turns Off Funding Spigot." *Modern Healthcare,* June 1981, pp. 106–7.

Gibson, Robert M. "National Health Expenditures, 1979." *Health Care Financing Review* 2, no. 1 (Summer 1980):1–36.

Glandon, Gerald, and Roberta Shapiro, eds. "Trends in Physicians' Incomes, Expenses and Fees 1970–1979." *Profile of Medical Practice, 1980.* Chicago: American Medical Association Center for Health Services Research and Development, 1980.

Grant, Dean. *How to Negotiate Physician Contracts.* Chicago: Teach 'Em Incorporated, 1979.

Greenspan, Nancy T., and Ronald J. Vogel. "Taxation and Its Effect Upon Public and Private Health Insurance and Medical Demand. *Health Care Financing Review,* Spring 1980, pp. 39–45.

Hallas, Gail Ghigna. "Why Nurses are Giving It Up." *RN Magazine,* July 1980, pp. 17–20.

Hammond, John. "Home Health Care Cost Effectiveness: An Overview of the Literature." *Public Health Reports* 94, no. 4 (July–August 1979): 305–11.

"Hospital Corporation of America Growth is 1,000–2,000 Beds Per Year." *Drug Research Reports—The Blue Sheet,* May 16, 1979, p. RN-3.

"House Unit Told Nurse Shortage May Affect Elders' Care." *Hospital Week* 16, no. 34 (August 1980):1.

Iglehart, John K. "HMOs An Idea Whose Time Has Come?" *National Journal,* February 25, 1978, pp. 311–14.

Illinois Hospital Association. *The Nursing Shortage in Illinois Hospitals.* September 1980.

Interstudy. *July 1980 Survey Results: HMO Enrollment and Utilization in the United States.* Excelsior, Minn.: Interstudy, November 1980.

"Investor-Owned Chain Hospitals Compete More." *Modern Healthcare,* August 1979 p. 24.

"Job Dissatisfaction Causes R.N. Shortage, Texas Study Shows." *American Journal of Nursing,* September 1980, pp. 1527–34.

Johnson, Donald E. "Mackey: For-Profit Systems Will Thrive." *Modern Healthcare,* August 1979, pp. 22–23.

_____, ed. "Multihospital System Survey, 1979." *Modern Healthcare,* April 1979, pp. 46–54.

_____, "Multihospital System Survey, 1980." *Modern Healthcare,* April 1980, pp. 57–98.

_____. "Multihospital System Survey, 1981." *Modern Healthcare,* April 1981, pp. 79–108.

Kalisch, Beatrice and Philip Kalisch. "Nursing Shortage—YES!" *American Journal of Nursing,* March 1979, pp. 469–80.

Katz, Barry P.; Michael S. Zdeb; and Gene D. Therriault. "Where People Die." *Public Health Reports* 94, no. 6 (November–December 1979): 522–27.

Kinkead, Gwen. "Humana's Hard Sell Hospitals." *Fortune,* November 17, 1980, pp. 68–81.

Kirchner, Merian. "Doctor Surplus: What 1990 Will Look Like." *Medical Economics,* September 29, 1980, pp. 54–62.

_____. "Professional Fee Survey." *Medical Economics,* October 13, 1980, pp. 207–23.

Koetting, Michael. *Nursing-Home Organization and Efficiency.* Lexington, Mass.: Lexington Books, 1980.

Koncel, Jerome A. "Private Health Insurance Looks at HMOs." *Hospitals,* August 16, 1980, pp. 137–42.

Kotler, Philip. *Marketing for Non-Profit Organizations.* Englewood Cliffs, N.J.: Prentice-Hall, 1975.

_____., and Sidney J. Levy. "Broadening the Concept of Marketing." *Journal of Marketing* 33 (January 1969).

Langford, Teddy, and Patricia Prescott. "Hospitals and Supplemental Nursing Agencies: An Uneasy Balance." *Journal of Nursing Administration,* November 1979, pp. 16–20.

LaViolette, Susan. "Collective Bargaining Given Funding, Priority Boost by ANA Delegates." *Modern Healthcare,* July 1980, p. 48.

_____. "Snowed Under by Regs, Hospitals Unbundle Services." *Modern Healthcare,* December 1980, pp. 52–54.

Lee, Josephine T., and Mary A. Stein. "Eliminating Duplication in Home Health Care for the Elderly: The Guale Projects." *Health and Social Work,* 1980, pp 29–36.

Levitt, Theodore. "Marketing Myopia." *Harvard Business Review,* July–August 1960.

Liang, Jersey; Eva Kahana; and Edmund Doherty. "Financial Well-Being Among the Aged: A Further Elaboration." *Journal of Gerontology,* 1980, pp. 409–19.

Littenberg, Benjamin, and Duncan Neuhauser. "To Hell with Economics?" *American Journal of Public Health,* April 1981, pp. 363–65.

Louis Harris and Associates. *American Attitudes Toward Health Maintenance Organizations.* Menlo Park, Calif.: The Henry J. Kaiser Family Foundation, July 1980.

Lublin, Joann S. "Severe Nurse Shortage Forces Some Hospitals to Close Beds or Units." *Wall Street Journal,* July 18, 1980, p. 1.

Luft, Harold S. "How do Health Maintenance Organizations Achieve Their 'Savings'?" *The New England Journal of Medicine* (June 15, 1978):1336–43.

_____. "Trends in Medical Care Costs: Do HMOs Lower the Rate of Growth?" *Medical Care,* January 1980, p. 1–16.

Mahoney, Anne Rankin. "Factors Affecting Physicians' Choice of Group or Independent Practice." *Inquiry,* June 1973, pp. 9–18.

Markel, William M. and Virginia B. Sinon. "The Hospice Concept." New York: American Cancer Society Professional Education Publications, 1978.

Mason, Scott. "Greater Access, Lower Costs with Multihospital Systems." *Hospital Financial Management,* May 1980, pp. 58–64.

_____. "The Multihospital Movement Defined." *Public Health Reports* 94, no. 5 (September–October 1979):446–52.

"M.D. Owned Insurance Firms Prove Successful." *U.S. Medicine,* December 1, 1978.

Meyer, Diane. "Grasp—Making the Most of Nursing Budgets." *Hospital Financial Management,* April 1980, pp. 32–36.

Miller, Alfred E.; Maria G. Miller; and Jonathan Adelman. "The Changing Urban-Suburban Distribution of Medical Practice in Large American Metropolitan Areas." *Medical Care* 16, no. 10 (October 1978):799–818.

Miller, Dulcy. "The Maturation of Long-Term Care." *Journal of Long-Term Care,* Spring 1979.

Moore, Florence M. "New Issues for In-Home Services." *Public Welfare,* Spring 1977, pp. 26–37.

Moore, Joan F., and Robert J. Grams. "Hospitals List Nurse Graduate Expectations." *Hospitals*, June 1, 1980, pp. 73–75.

Morell, James A., and Peter G. Rogan. "Hospital Based Physician Compensation Concepts." *Topics in Health Care Financing*, "Physician Compensation," edited by David Pieroni. Spring 1978, pp. 11–25.

Morrow, Gloria, narrator. "Conference on Nurse Recruitment and Retention." *American Health Care Association Journal*, May 1980, pp. 3–9.

Moses, Evelyn, and Aleda Roth. "Nursepower." *American Journal of Nursing*, October 1979, pp. 1745–56.

Moss, Frank E., and Val J. Halamandaris. *Too Old, Too Sick, Too Bad—Nursing Homes in America*. Germantown, Md.: Aspen Systems Corporation, 1977.

"Multihospital Chains Add Services." *Modern Healthcare*, August 1980, p. 42.

National Association of Nurse Recruiters. *R.N. Hospital Vacancy Survey, January 1980*. Pitman, N.J.: National Association of Nurse Recruiters, 1980.

National League for Nursing. *Nurse Career Pattern Study Baccalaureate Degree, Nurses Ten Years After Graduation*. New York: National League for Nursing, March 1979.

Neely, Marvin F. "Cooperative Recruitment: One Approach." *Hospitals*, July 1, 1980, pp. 70–71.

"A New Licensing Exam for Nurses." Interview with Eileen McQuaid and Phyllis Sheil. *American Journal of Nursing*, April 1980, pp. 723–26.

Norris, John R. "The Acute Hospital-Chronic Hospital Affiliation: A Comparison of Length of Stay of Chronic Patients in Affiliated and Non-affiliated Acute Hospitals." *Medical Care* 9, no. 6 (November–December 1971):479–86.

"Nurse Recruiting Widens." *New York Times*, October 31, 1979.

"The Nurse Shortage: There's a Long Road Ahead." *Hospitals*, May 1, 1980, pp. 63–64.

"Nursing Homes Hit Hardest by RN Shortage." *American Journal of Nursing*, October 1980, pp. 1720–44.

"Nursing Is Not a Woman's Profession." *RN Magazine*, April 1980.

"Nursing Shortage." *Washington Report on Health Legislation*, August 27, 1980.

O'Keefe, James J., III. "Survival of Hospitals in America: More Than First Aid is Needed. *L & H Perspective*, Spring–Summer 1980, pp. 3–5.

O'Keefe, Niki. "Choosing a Nurse Recruiter." *Hospitals*, July 1, 1980, pp. 74–75.

Osterweis, Marian, and Daphne Szmuszkovic Champagne. "The U.S. Hospice Movement: Issues in Development." *American Journal of Public Health* 69, no. 5, (May 1979):492–96.

Owens, Arthur. "Doctor Surplus: Where Things Stand Now." *Medical Economics*, September 29, 1980, pp. 63–80.

Perkins, Roy. "The Physicians' View of the Hospital: A Love-Hate Relationship." *The Hospital Medical Staff: Selected Readings, 1972–1978*. Chicago: American Hospital Association, 1977.

Personett, Judith D., and Mary A. Boyle. "Abuse, Poor Image Causes Shortage." *Modern Healthcare*, July 1980, p. 92.

"Physician Hospital Conflict: The Hospital Staff Privileges Controversy in New York." *Cornell Law Journal* 60 (1975):1075–1104.

"Physician Influence: Applying Noerr Pennington to the Medical Profession." *Duke Law Journal* 1978, no. 2 (May 1978).

"Physicians Locate Where Benefits Best." *Modern Healthcare*, March 1979, p. 34.

Pollak, William. "Utilization of Alternative Care Settings by the Elderly." In *Community Planning for an Aging Society: Designing Services and Facilities*, edited by M. Powell Lawton, Robert J. Newcomer, and Thomas O. Byerts. Stroudsburg, Pa.: Dowden, Hutchingson and Ross, Inc., 1976, pp. 106–27.

Prybil, Lawrence D. "Provision of Long-Term Care Services by Community Hospitals in Virginia." *Hospital and Health Services Administration*, Fall 1980, pp. 80–102.

Reinhardt, Uwe E. *Physician Productivity and the Demand for Health Manpower*. Cambridge, Mass.: Ballinger Publishing, 1975.

Relman, Arnold S. "The New Medical Industrial Complex." *New England Journal of Medicine,* October 23, 1980, pp. 963–70.

"Review Responsibilities for HSAs." *Today in Health Planning* 2, no. 20 (May 16, 1980).

Roodman, Richard D. "Physicians' Office Condos—A Unique Approach to Capital Development." *Health Financing Management,* September 1980, pp. 20–26.

Rottkamp, Barbara. "Survey of Nurse Attitudes Toward Professional Nursing Practice." *Journal of Nursing Education* 19, no. 5 (May 1980):32–38.

Scanlon, William J. "A Theory of the Nursing Home Market." *Inquiry,* Spring 1980, pp. 25–41.

Schroeder, Steven M. D.; Jonathan A. Showstack, M.P.H.; and H. Edith Roberts. "Frequency and Clinical Description of High Cost Patients in 17 Acute Care Hospitals." *The New England Journal of Medicine* (June 7, 1979):1306–9.

Schwartz, Michael; Suzanne Griesez Martin; Deborah D'Arpa Cooper; Greta M. Jung; Bernadette J. Whalen; and Joseph Blackburn. "The Effect of a Thirty Per Cent Reduction in Physician Fees on Medicaid Surgery Rates in Massachusetts." *American Journal of Public Health* 71, no. 4 (April 1981): 370–75.

Schwartz, William; Joseph Newhouse; Bruce Bennett; and Albert Williams. "The Changing Geographic Distribution of Board Certified Physicians." *The New England Journal of Medicine,* October 30, 1980, pp. 1032–38.

_____. *The Changing Geographic Distribution of Board Certified Physicians.* Santa Monica, Calif.: The Rand Corporation, October 1980.

"Senate Committee Approves Resolution to Study Nurse Shortage." *Legislative Reporter* 13, no. 25 (June 13, 1980).

Sengelaub, Sr. Mary Maurita. "Catholic Health Care Systems: A Sign of the Times." In Montague Brown and Barbara McCool, *Multihospital Systems: Strategies for Organization and Management.* Rockville, Md.: Aspen Systems Corporation, 1980.

Seybolt, John, and Duane Walker. "Attitude Survey Proves to be a Powerful Tool for Reversing Turnover." *Hospitals,* May 1, 1980, pp. 77–78.

Sharfstein, Steven, and Harry Clark. "Why Psychiatry is a Low-Paid Medical Specialty." *American Journal of Psychiatry,* July 1980, pp. 831–33.

"60% of all Baccalaureate Degree RNs Are Employed." *Drug Research Reports—The Blue Sheet,* April 4, 1979.

Sloan, Frank A.; Jerry Cromwell; and Janet B. Mitchell. *Private Physicians and Public Programs.* Lexington, Mass.: Lexington Books, 1978.

Smyer, Michael A. "The Differential Usage of Services by Impaired Elderly." *Journal of Gerontology* 35, no. 2, (1980): 249–55.

Somers, Anne. "Rethinking Health Policy for the Elderly: A Six Point Program." *Inquiry,* Spring 1980, pp. 3–17.

"Sources of Funding for Construction." *Hospitals,* February 16, 1979, p. 63.

Steinwald, Bruce. "Hospital Based Physicians: Current Issues and Descriptive Evidence." *Health Care Financing Review,* Summer 1980, pp. 63–75.

"Survival of Hospices Depends on Insurers." *Modern Healthcare,* November 1979, p. 58.

"Symposium on the Antitrust Laws and the Health Services Industry." *Duke Law Journal* 1978, no. 2 (May 1978):543–85.

"Task Force Sets 1982 Target Date for Credentialing Center." *American Journal of Nursing,* August 1980, p. 1394.

Taylor, Elworth. "Survey Shows Who Is Sharing Which Services." *Hospitals* 53 (September 16, 1979).

"Unique Ad Strategy Increases Use of Sunrise Hospital on Weekends." *Federation of American Hospitals Review* 10, no. 3 (June 1977).

United States Department of Commerce, Bureau of the Census. *Construction Reports.* Washington, D.C., October 1980.

United States Department of Health and Human Services, Health Care Financing Administration. *Costs Incurred for Patient Solicitation (Unallowable Cost of Advertising).* Washington, D.C., 1979.

_____. United States Department of Health and Human Services, Office of Research, Demonstrations and Statistics, Health Care Financing Administration. *Medicare: Participating Health Facilities, 1979.* Washington, D.C., 1979.

_____. *Medicare Program Statistics Report—Utilization of Home Health Services, 1977.* Washington, D.C., 1979.

_____. *Medicare: Use of Home Health Services, 1978.* Washington, D.C., 1979.

United States Department of Health and Human Services, Public Health Service, Office of Health Research, Statistics and Technology, *Advancedata, 1978 Summary: National Ambulatory Medical Care Survey.* Washington, D.C., April 23, 1980, no. 60.

_____. Report to the Congress. *Home Health Services Under Titles XVIII, XIX and XX.* April 1979.

_____. Public Health Service Office of Health Research, Statistics and Technology. "Who Initiates Visits to a Physician?" Data Previews, National Health Care Expenditures Study, September 1980.

United States Department of Health and Human Services, Vital and Health Statistics, National Center for Health Statistics. *The National Nursing Home Survey: 1977 Summary for the United States.* Series 13, no. 43, July 1979.

United States Department of Health and Human Services. *Report of the Graduate Medical Education National Advisory Committee to the Secretary.* September 1980, Vol. 1.

United States Department of Health and Human Services, Office of Inspector General Audit Agency. *Report on Need for More Restrictive Policy and Procedures Covering Medicare Reimbursement for Medical Services Provided by Hospital based Physicians.* Audit Control Number 06–02001.

United States Department of Health and Human Services, Public Health Service, Office of Health Maintenance Organizations. *National HMO Census 1980.* June 30, 1980, DHHS Publication no. (PHS) 80–501159.

United States Department of Health and Human Services, Public Health Service Office of Health Research, Statistics and Technology, *Health United States 1980, 1979, 1978.*

United States Department of Labor, Bureau of Labor Statistics. *Employment and Earnings United States, 1909–1978.* Bulletin no. 1312–11.

_____. *Employment Projections for the 1980s.*

_____. *Supplement to Employment and Earnings: Revised Establishment Data, 1980.*

United States General Accounting Office, Comptroller General Report to the Congress. *Are Enough Physicians of the Right Type Trained in the United States?* 1978.

_____. *Entering A Nursing Home Costly Implications for Medicaid and the Elderly.* November 26, 1979, PAD–80–12.

_____. *Health Maintenance Organizations Can Help Control Health Care Costs.* May 6, 1980.

University of Chicago Graduate Program in Hospital Administration and Center for Health Administration Studies, Graduate School of Business. Proceedings of the Twenty First Annual Symposium on Hospital Affairs. *Changing the Behavior of the Physician: A Management Perspective.* June 1979.

Vraciu, Robert, and Howard S. Zuckerman. "Legal and Financial Constraints on the Development and Growth of Multiple Hospital Arrangements." *Health Care Management Review,* 4, no. 10 (Winter 1979):39–47.

Wald, Florence; Zelda Foster; and Henry J. Wald. "The Hospice Movement as a Health Care Reform. *Nursing Outlook,* March 1980.

Wan, Thomas; William G. Weissert; and Barbara Livieratos. "Geriatric Day Care and Homemaker Services: An Experimental Study." *Journal of Gerontology* 35, no. 2 (1980):256–73.

Wandelt, Mabel A., Patricia A. Pierce; and Robert R. Widdowson. "Why Nurses Leave Nursing and What Can Be Done About It." *American Journal of Nursing,* January 1981, pp. 72–77.

Way, Peter O.; Lynn E. Jensen; and Louis J. Goodman. "Foreign Medical Graduates and the Issue of Substantial Disruption of Medical Services." *The New England Journal of Medicine*, October 5, 1978, pp. 745–51.

Weissert, William G. "Costs of Adult Day Care: A Comparison to Nursing Homes." *Inquiry* (March 1978):10–19.

_____.; Thomas T. H. Wan; Barbara Livieratos; and Julius Pellegrino. "Cost Effectiveness of Homemaker Services for the Chronically Ill." *Inquiry* (Fall 1980):230–43.

Wunderman, Lorna E. *Physician Distribution and Medical Licensure in the U.S., 1978*. Chicago: American Medical Association Center for Health Research and Development, 1979.

Zukerman, Howard S. "Multi-Institutional Systems: Promise and Performance." *Inquiry*, Winter 1979, pp. 291–314.

Index

A

ABT Associates, 118
Aftercare, 18; *see also* Home health care;
    Hospices; *and* Nursing homes
  coordination of services; *see also*
    Triage Incorporated
  hospital-based programs
    day care (geriatric), 72
    home health care, 73
  physician participation, 70, 73
Alt, Joyce, 193
Alternative delivery systems; *see* Health
  maintenance organizations
Ambulances; *see* Hospitals,
  transportation systems
Ambulatory care programs, freestanding,
  221; *see also* Flashner, Bruce, M.D.;
  Hospitals, feeder systems; *and*
  Wayne State Medical School, Health
  Care Institute
  ambulatory surgery centers, 38, 40–42
  kidney dialysis centers, 44–45
  urgent care centers, 42–43
American Hospital Association
  Guide to the Health Care Field, 7, 10,
    120

Hospital Panel Survey, 1980, 14
Hospital Research and Education
  Trust, 108
Hospital Shared Services Participation
  Profile (1978), 129
Hospital Statistics, 53, 55
American Medical Association, 33, 35
  HMO survey, 82–83, 87
  physician data surveys, 27–30, 35
American Medical International, Inc.,
  114, 121
American Nursing Association, 186
Anderson, Odin, evolution of health care
  industry, 102–5
Arthur Young and Company, 64, 66
ARA Services, Inc., 63
Arthur Young and Company, 64, 66
Atkinson, J. Graham, 12

B

Bailey, R. M., 36
Bates, Mary, 193
Bays, Carson, 117–18
Bennett, B. W., 32
Biles, Brian, 12
BioServices; *see* Rush Presbyterian St.
  Lukes

Blue Cross/Blue Shield Insurance
Companies, 14, 20, 70, 82, 84, 94, 113
Brown, Montague, 128–29
multihospital system survey, 108

C

Caldwell, George, 155, 157–58; *see also*
Lutheran General Hospital
Calhoun, Gary, 190
California Medicaid Program (MediCal),
20, 40
Campbell, James, M.D., 149, 151–53; *see
also* Rush Presbyterian St. Lukes
Medical Center
Carter administration, 9
Certificate of Need; *see* Government
regulations
Chandler, Alfred; *see also* Corporate
organization
evolution of corporate organization,
97–101, 120–22
Chicago Medical Society, 35
Clark, Robert, 116–17
Cleveland Clinic, 137, 174
Coelen, Craig, 118
Competition
economic, effects on health care
industry, 1, 13–14, 16, 18–19, 77,
201–4
freestanding units and hospitals, 42, 44
hospitals and physicians, 46
physicians, 32
and freestanding units, 43
regional and national management
firms, 125, 127
Contract management, participation of
investor owned firms, 63, 114–15
regional nonprofits, 126–27
Cook County Hospital of Chicago, 114,
151, 153
Cooperider, Fran, 198
Corporate organization; *see also*
Hospitals, corporate restructuring
application to hospital industry, 102–
5, 136, 203, 219–20
consolidation, 99
integration, 99–100
Corpus, Tita, 189
Criles, George, M.D., 167
Cunningham, Frances, 87

D

Daley, Richard, 153
Davis, James E., 38
Demand
hospital services, 22–23
nurses, 187–88

Demand—*Cont.*
nursing home services, 53, 61
physician services, 26–32
Derzon, Robert, 127
Detmer, Donald E., 38
Dietz, Joan, 61
DiPaolo, Vincent, 62–63
Discovery effect; *see* Home health care,
cost studies
Doctors Emergency Officenter; *see* Bruce
Flashner, M.D.
Donabedian, Avedis, 65–66
Donovan, Lynn, 191, 194
Drucker, Peter, marketing concept, 2, 216
Duke Law Review, 169
Dunlop, Burton, 53, 55, 58–59

E

Eastman Kodak, 3
Elderly population; *see also* Health care
expenditures *and* Nursing homes
statistics, 50–52
Ellwood, Paul, 85, 93
Enthoven, Alain C., 12–13, 78, 90
Ernst, Richard, 35
Evangelical Hospital Association, 124

F

Federation of American Hospitals, 113,
116, 120
Feeder systems; *see* Hospitals, feeder
systems
Fisher, Charles, 50
Flashner, Bruce, M.D., 43
Ford, Henry, Hospital of Detroit, 124
Forster, Zelda, 69
Fralic, Maryann, RN, 184, 188
Freestanding ambulatory care programs;
see Ambulatory care programs,
freestanding
Fries, James, M.D., 22

G

Gabel, Jon R., 26, 163
General Accounting Office, 61
General Electric, Incorporated, 70
Gibson, Robert, 7, 9, 33, 119
Gilmore, Maryann, 193
Glandon, Gerald, 28, 36
Good Samaritan Hospital of Phoenix; *see*
Samaritan Health Service
Government regulations
Aid to the Aged, Blind and Disabled
Programs, 58
Certificate of Need, 11–12, 60, 113, 177,
180, 222
Federal HMO Act of 1973, 85

Government regulations—*Cont.*
  Health Care Financing Administration, 71
    demonstration projects; *see* Triage Incorporated
    Diagnosis-based Reimbursement Group (DRG), 20, 215
    Professional Standards Review Organization (PSRO), 16
  Health Planning and Resource Development Act of 1975 (PL 93–641), 11; *see also* Health Systems Agencies
    1977 Amendments, 177
  Hospital Survey and Construction Act (Hill-Burton), 10–11, 102
  Life Safety Code, 58
  Old Age Assistance, 58
  Partnership in Health Act of 1966, 11
Graduate Medical Education National Advisory Committee, 30, 208–9; *see also* Physician, distribution
Grant, Dean, 167, 171–72

H

Hammond, John, 65
Harris, Louis, and Associates, 83–86, 89
Harvard Business Review, 3
Health care expenditures
  aggregate amounts, 7, 9
  National Entitlement Programs, 19, 21–22, 50, 52, 56, 64–65, 70, 177
  patient pay, 19, 56, 70, 201
Health Care Financing Administration (HCFA), 71
Health maintenance organizations, 18; *see also* Hospitals, feeder systems *and* Kaiser Permanente Health Care Program
  comparisons to fee for service systems, 78–79, 81, 86–87
  consumer attitudes, 83–89
  cost study data, 81, 88
  employer participation, 85, 88, 90
  enrollment data, 83–85, 88–89, 93
  hospital utilization rates, 81–82, 89, 92–93
  management arrangements, 78–79
  physician participation, 79–80, 91
  salary arrangements, 80
  variations
    hospital-based HMOs, 93–94
    Independent Practice Associations, 79–82, 87–88, 91, 94
    insurer owned, 84, 94–95.
    prepaid group practice, 79, 82, 87
    primary care networks, 80

Health Systems Agencies, 11, 221–22
  Central Arizona Health Systems Agency, 39
Hillhaven Corporation; *see* National Medical Enterprises
Home health care
  cost studies, 65–66
  efficacy, 68
  hospital-based, 66
  investor owned agencies, 66
  range of services, 64
  reimbursement, 65, 69
    regulations, 64, 66
  respite care, 68
Hospices; *see also* Saunders, Cicely, M.D., *and* Saint Christopher's Hospice
  description of services, 69
  insurability, 70
Hospital Affiliates International; *see* INA Corporation
Hospital associations, 221
  California Hospital Association, 186
  Illinois Hospital Association, 185, 194–95
Hospital Corporation of America, 119, 121
Hospital management firms; *see* Investor owned hospital management firms
Hospitals
  administrators' role
    maintaining utilization, 172
    management of hospital, 173, 204
    physician compensation, 163, 165–66, 173
    productivity, 170, 220–21
    recruitment, 171
  ancillary services, 38
    billing arrangements, 165–67
  bed supply, 11–12
  corporate restructuring; *see also* Lutheran General Hospital *and* Rush Presbyterian St. Lukes Medical Center
    effect on revenues, 154–55, 159
    incentives to restructure, 154, 158–59, 203
  cost containment, 12–13
  educational programs, 144–45
  feeder systems
    disadvantages, 141–42, 144
    function, 17, 136, 180
    variations
      emergency rooms, 42, 139
      health maintenance organizations, 142
      physician office buildings, 139–40

Hospitals—*Cont.*
  feeder systems—*Cont.*
    variations—*Cont.*
      private physician practice, 137,
        142, 178–79, 207
      satellite hospitals, 141–42
  medical staff
    closed staffs, 168–70
    productivity issues, 170, 220
    recruitment, 170, 211
  outpatient departments; *see also*
      Hospitals, corporate restructuring
    alternative substructures, 177
    cost effectiveness, 175
    reimbursement principles, 176–77
  physician compensation
    economic conflicts with hospital, 167,
      172
    fee-for-service system, 64, 166, 175
    guaranteed minimum income, 166
    hospital based physicians, 164–65,
      172
    percentage arrangements, 164–66
    salaried arrangements, 138, 163, 165,
      167, 174
  transportation systems
    aircraft; *see* University of Iowa
      Hospitals and Clinics *and*
      Samaritan Health Service of
      Phoenix
    ambulances, 148
  trustees, 162, 170–71, 173, 179, 222
  utilization rates, 6, 14–16, 37, 214
  surgical utilization, 38, 213

I

IBM Corporation, 3
INA Corporation, 63, 121
Independent Practice Associations; *see*
  Health maintenance organizations
Intermountain Health Service; *see*
  Multihospital systems, nonprofit
  systems, regional *and* Scott Parker
Internal Revenue Service, 179
Interstudy, Incorporated, 18, 83
Investor owned hospital management
  firms; *see also* Multihospital systems
  foreign markets, 116, 119
  growth strategies, 120–22
  management policies, 119, 122
  market share, 116
  profit controversies, 116–19

J–K

Johnson, Donald, 123
Johnson Foundation, Robert Wood, 42

Journal of Marketing, 3
Kaiser Permanente Medical Care
  Program, 18, 78, 81, 84–85, 123
Kalisch, Beatrice and Philip, 184, 189
Keogh plan, 34
Koetting, Michael, 62–63
Kotler, Philip, nonprofit marketing, 3–4

L

Langford, Tedd, 194
Lee, Josephine, 61
Levitt, Theodore, 3
Levy, Sidney J., 4
Lewin, and Associates, 117
Lewin Lawrence, 127
Livieratos, Barbara, 68
Long-term care; *see* Nursing homes
Luft, Harold S., 81–82
Lutheran General Hospital
  components
    foundation for Human Ecology, 157
    Lutheran Institute of Human
      Ecology, 155
    Parkside Foundation, 157
    Parkside Medical Services
      Corporation, 157
  organization, 157–58

M

Mahoney, Anne Ranking, 26, 35–36
Market audit—hospitals, 205, 209, 218,
  222
  consumer attitudes, 209, 218
  patient origin, 207, 218, 221
  patient satisfaction, 216–17, 219
  payer mix, 214–15
  physician practice data, 206–7, 212–13,
    221
  physician-to-population ratios, 208–9,
    211
Marketing, health care; *see* Peter
  Drucker, marketing concept *and*
  Philip Kotler, nonprofit marketing
Massachusetts General Hospital, 177
Mayo Clinic, 137, 174
McDonalds, 3
Medical staff arrangements; *see*
  Hospitals, medical staff
Medical underservice; *see* Physicians,
  distribution
Meyer, Diane, 198
Mitchell, Janet B., 26–27, 35
Modern Healthcare, 45, 70, 107, 122–23
Morell, James A., 165–66
Moses, Evelyn, 186
Mount Sinai Hospital of Chicago, 177

Multihospital affiliations
consortia, 130–31
shared services, 130
Multihospital systems; *see also* Contract
management
antitrust issues, 131
corporate organization, 108, 124–25, 132
investor owned systems, capital
financing, 108–10, 112–13
market share, 107–8
nonprofit systems, 127–28
organizational arrangements, 108,
110
nonprofit systems, regional, 110, 122–
23, 125; *see also* Evangelical
Hospital Association; Henry Ford
Hospital of Detroit; Intermountain
Health Service; Lutheran General
Hospital; Rush Presbyterian St.
Lukes Medical Center; Samaritan
Health Service of Phoenix; *and*
Sisters of Mercy Health
Corporation
capital financing, 127–28

N

National Association of Nurse Recruiters,
184, 196
National Institute for Occupational
Safety and Health, 190
National League of Nursing, 184, 187, 189
National Medical Enterprises, 63, 121
Neely, Marvin F., 196
New England Journal of Medicine, 22, 116
Newhouse, J. P., 32
Northwestern University, 3
Nurses
career patterns, 189
job satisfaction, 191, 193–94
labor force participation, 186–87
recruitment, 196, 199
registries, 194–95
retention strategies, 197–99
salaries, 191, 196
shortage data, 184, 187
staffing practices, 189, 197
stress factors, 190–91, 193
Nursing education, 192, 198
enrollment data, 187
Nursing homes
investor owned, 59, 61–62
efficiency; *see* Koetting, Michael
Medicaid and Medicare
reimbursement, 50, 55–60
quality of care, 60, 62
revenues, 56

Nursing homes—*Cont.*
statistics, 52–53
utilization, 53–55, 59–60

O–P

Orkand Corporation, 42
Owens, Arthur, 29, 33
Parker, Scott, 125; *see also* Intermountain
Health Service
Patient satisfaction; *see* Market audit
Perkins, Roy, 167
Peter Principle; *see* Nurses, job
satisfaction
Physicians
activity levels, 27, 29–30
distribution, 31–32
foreign medical graduates, 31–32, 207–
8
practice
corporate practice of medicine, 33–
35
fee-for-service, 26–27
group practice, 32, 35–36
income trends, 26–30, 36
incorporation, 33–34
practice patterns, 26, 29, 35, 212
solo practice, 26, 32, 36
specialty requirements, 31, 210–11, 223;
see also Graduate Medical
Education National Advisory
Committee
PL 93–641; *see* Government regulations
Polaroid Corporation, 3
Pollok, William, 53–54
Prescott, Patricia A., 194
Proctor & Gamble, 3

R

Reagan administration, 12
Redisch, Michael, 26, 163
Reinhardt, Uwe, 26, 35
Relman, Arnold, M.D., 116
Respite care; *see* Home health care
Revlon, Incorporated, 3
RN Magazine, 184
Roemer effect; *see* Hospitals, bed supply
Rogan, Peter C., 165–66
Roth, Aleda, 186
Rush Presbyterian St. Lukes Medical
Center, 177–78
components
Anchor HMO, 150–51
BioServices, 152
Bowman Geriatrics Center, 151, 153
Miles Square Health Center, 150–51
Rush Medical College, 149, 151
Sheridan Road Pavilion, 152

Rush Presbyterian St. Lukes Medical
    Center—*Cont.*
    goals of system, 149
    health personnel training, 150
    regional affiliations, 124, 149, 151
    voluntary hospital system, 152

S

SAFECO Insurance Company, 80
Saint Christopher's Hospice, 69; *see also*
    Hospices
Samaritan Health Service of Phoenix, 44,
    123, 147
    Good Samaritan Hospital, 41, 124, 147
Saunders, Cicely, M.D., 69; *see also*
    Hospices
Scanlon, William, 52, 59–60, 63
Schramm, Carl J., 12
Schwartz, W. B., 32
Sengelaub, Mary, 123
Shapiro, Roberta, 28, 36
Shared services; *see* Multihospital
    affiliations
Sisters of Mercy Health Corporation, 123
Sloan, Frank A., 26–27, 35
Somers, Anne, 50–51
Stein, Mary, 61
Steinwald, Bruce, 164
Sullivan, Daniel, 118
Surveys; *see* Market audit

T

Taxation
    hospitals, tax-exempt status, 117, 179
    physician practice, 33–34
Taylor, Elworth, 107, 130
Triage Incorporated, 71–72
Tulane University Medical Center, 121

U

U.S. Department of Commerce, Census
    Bureau, 55, 218
U.S. Department of Health and Human
    Services, 30, 186
    health care in United States, 1979, 1980,
        7, 62
    National HMO Census, 1980, 81
    National Nursing Home Survey, 62
United States Steel Corporation, 99; *see
    also* Corporate organization
University of Chicago Hospitals and
    Clinics, 35, 74, 208–9
University of Illinois Medical Center, 153
University of Iowa Hospitals and Clinics,
    147

V–Y

Visiting Nurse Association, 66
Vladeck, Bruce, 60
Wald, Florence, 69
Wald, Henry, 69
Wan, Thomas, 68
Watt, J. Michael, 127
Wayne State University Medical School,
    130
    Health Care Institute, 131
Weissert, William, 61, 68, 73
Western Interstate Commission for
    Higher Education, 187
Westinghouse Corporation, 70
Williams, A. P., 32
Williamson, John, 87
Young, Arthur, and Company, 64, 66

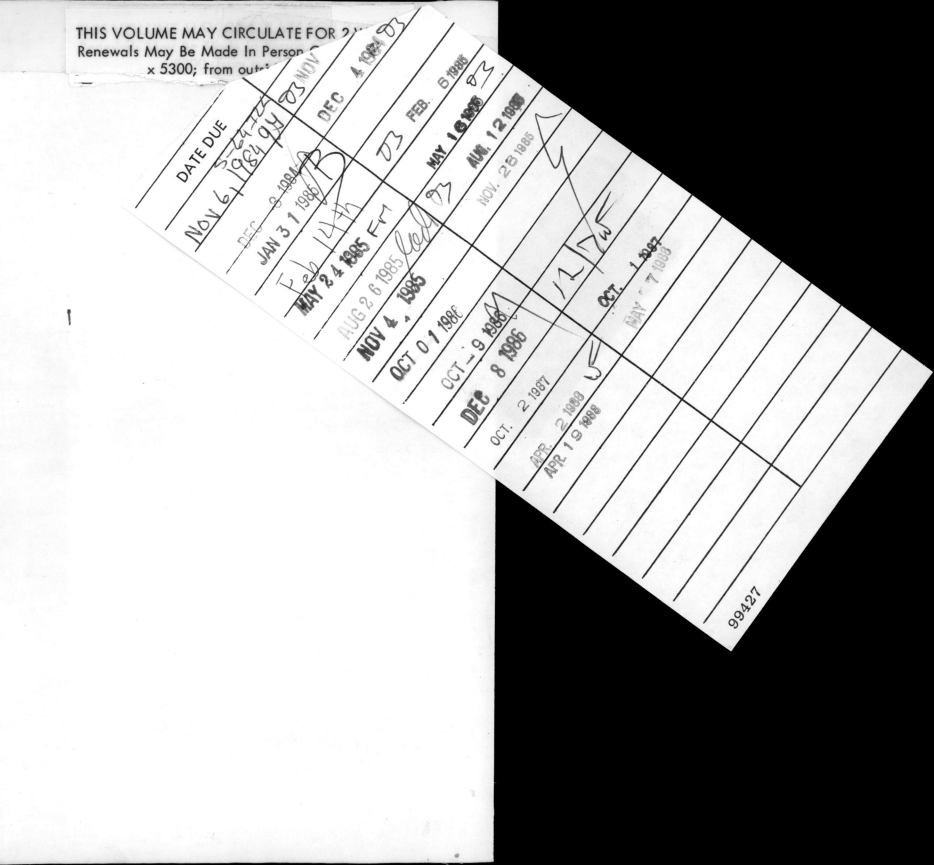